Crohn's Conspiracy

by "Steve"

Prepress & Editing

by

Page Telegram Services, et al.

ISBN: 979-8-9990071-8-6

Bulk Orders Available:
CrohnsConspiracy.com

info@CrohnsConspiracy.com

GRATITUDES

Gratitude to the following people for which this book and my journey to recovery would not have been possible: Jason Page, Nick Scuba, Nic Sementa, Two (TSK), Dr. Maria, Dr. Cohen (surgeon), Dr. Saporta (GI), Dr Zanneti (HBO) my mother, my family, our book cover designer Marty (a good friend) & talented artist.

DEDICATION

To those who have endured the weight of Crohn's disease and the shadow of Mycobacterium avium paratuberculosis (MAP) disease, this is for you your resilience speaks louder than the silence of an industry that has too often looked away.

You've faced relentless pain, uncertainty and the frustration of treatments that patch symptoms while the root cause festers, unaddressed. You've navigated a system that sometimes dismisses your struggle, offering bandages for wounds that demand deeper healing. Yet, you persist through flareups, fatigue and the quiet battles no one sees.

This dedication honors your courage to keep searching for answers, to question the status quo and to hold onto hope when the path feels impossibly steep. You are not defined by the blind spots of medicine but by your unyielding spirit in the face of them.

May your voices rise, your stories spark change and your suffering pave the way for a future where the root causes of diseases like Crohn's and MAP are no longer ignored, but confronted with the clarity and care you deserve. You are seen, you are heard and you are not alone in this battle against this medical industrial complex.

AUTHOR'S DISCLAIMER

As I present this work to the public, I feel compelled to affirm my state of mind and purpose with unequivocal clarity. I, known publicly as just "Steve," am of sound mind and body, driven by a commitment to explore challenging truths and foster meaningful discourse. I am not, nor have I ever been, suicidal; my passion for this project stems from a desire to illuminate, not to self-destruct. The ideas contained herein are the product of rigorous inquiry and a belief in the power of transparency to effect change nothing more, nothing less.

Given the controversial nature of this book, I am aware that it may provoke strong reactions, misinterpretations, or even unfounded speculation about my well-being. To preempt such narratives, I state plainly: any suggestion of self-harm or coercion in relation to my life or this work would be categorically false and contrary to the evidence of my character and intentions, as known to those closest to me. My aim is to contribute to a broader conversation, not to invite personal peril. I entrust this record to my readers and ask that it be judged on its merits, not overshadowed by fabricated doubts.

TABLE OF CONTENTS

III. PREFACE

Why This Book?

"Health is Wealth"

My name is Steve, and for the last forty years, my life has been a battleground for a disease I never chose, subjected to treatments I never fully understood, and entangled in a system that seems more invested in managing my illness than curing it. This book is not just my story it's an exposé, a revelation of the patterns I've uncovered through a lifetime of grappling with Crohn's disease. It merges the insights of two volumes into a single, comprehensive exploration of a medical system that often prioritizes profit over healing.

Crohn's has been my unrelenting shadow. My mother suffered from it, and my father passed away from stomach cancer at the age of 26, leaving me with a haunting question: was I genetically doomed, or is there something more sinister at play? Over decades of treatments, I became a reluctant lab rat in a grand medical experiment, enduring countless surgeries, navigating an ever-shifting pharmaceutical regimen, and scouring data from around the world spanning the UK, Australia, India, Canada, and beyond for answers. What I found was a web of inconsistencies, suppressed truths, and a healthcare industry that thrives on perpetuating chronic illness.

At first, I trusted the prevailing medical narrative: Crohn's is genetic, incurable, and best managed through lifelong dependence on medication. I wanted to believe the experts, to trust that medicine was working in my best interest. But patterns emerged that didn't add up. Why did my condition often worsen with each new pharmaceutical "breakthrough"? Why were dietary factors dismissed when I could feel their impact firsthand? Why did the industry seem so invested in keeping patients like me on a never-ending cycle of treatment rather than pursuing a cure? And why were promising alternative approaches like anti-Mycobacterium avium subspecies paratuberculosis (MAP) therapy, hyperbaric oxygen therapy, or cannabis routinely sidelined, buried under regulatory red tape or outright erased from public access?

This book is the culmination of four decades of observation, experience, and relentless inquiry. I've been prescribed a cocktail of pharmaceuticals corticosteroids, Humira, Remicade, Cimzia, Metronidazole, Imuran, and more witnessing the revolving door of medical trends, from steroids to immunosuppressants to biologics, each promising relief but often leaving me with more questions than answers. Through exhaustive research, I've uncovered alarming truths about the pharmaceutical and food industries and their roles in perpetuating chronic illness. The same organizations that shape dietary guidelines like the food pyramid we all grew up with are often backed by corporations profiting from the very diseases these diets exacerbate. I was raised on dairy, believing it to be essential, despite mounting evidence of its inflammatory effects. Meanwhile, data and studies I relied on, particularly those related to milk and MAP, have vanished from public access since I accessed them between 2015 and 2023, as if the truth is being systematically erased.

This expanded edition delves deeper into the Crohn's conspiracy, exploring the role of Mycobacterium avium subspecies paratuberculosis (MAP) and the groundbreaking work of pioneers like Robert Koch, Hermann Johne, Laurence Frothingham, Thomas Borody, R. Chiodini, and J. Aitken. It examines the inertia surrounding MAP research, exemplified by efforts like RedHill Biopharma, and exposes how Crohn's disease has become a profit machine for an industry projected to grow from $20 billion in 2022 to $36 billion by 2033, driven by key players like AbbVie, Pfizer, and Takeda. I uncover hidden treatments, erased data, and the sinister legacy of corporate giants like Bayer, alongside the manipulative "Got Milk?" campaigns of the 1990s, which obscured the inflammatory risks of dairy. The contributions of researchers like Borody, whose health is reportedly declining, are at risk of being lost, making it urgent to preserve their work for future generations.

We are in an era where long-suppressed truths are beginning to surface. Growing skepticism toward Big Pharma, coupled with revelations about harmful additives, pesticides like glyphosate, artificial dyes, and preservatives, points to a broader system of control over public health one driven more by profit than by patient well-being. Researchers and patients are reevaluating the interplay of genetics, environment, and lifestyle, questioning whether Crohn's is truly a purely genetic condition or a product of dietary influences, environmental toxins, and corporate priorities. This shift demands a new paradigm that prioritizes root causes over symptom management.

This book is not just about my journey; it's about shedding light on a healthcare system that thrives on industry-driven medicine. Crohn's is just one example of how chronic illnesses are managed rather than eradicated. I want readers to ask questions, seek alternative perspectives, and understand that modern medicine, while powerful, is also a business one that often profits from perpetual treatment rather than true healing.

Because health isn't just wealth it's power. And it's time we reclaim it.

THE FIRST 10 YEARS

A Childhood of Pain and Discovery

Born in Chicago in early 1980's, I spent most of my early years in the North side of the city. My heritage was deeply rooted in my Greek ancestry, and although I mostly grew up in the United States, I also lived in Europe for a time as a child. My early years were filled with challenges that no child should have to endure, from health struggles to family hardships, each leaving an indelible mark on my life. From birth, my health was fragile. Within my first month, doctors noticed something alarming I was passing blood in my stool. Concerned, they immediately removed all dairy products from my diet, a decision that, in hindsight, was crucial. However, I wouldn't learn the full extent of this dietary necessity until I was in my twenties. Had I known earlier, I might have been able to prevent years of pain and suffering.

Growing up, I experienced relentless joint pain and inflammation. By the time I was four, I became increasingly aware of the discomfort, and by five, I was undergoing X-rays and medical exams in an attempt to identify the problem. Despite my persistent pain, the scans never revealed any fractures or abnormalities, leaving doctors to dismiss my condition as mere "growing pains." But I knew better something was deeply wrong.

At the same time, my family life was unraveling. My stepfather, who had been in my life for three years, tragically passed away in a fatal accident. The loss was overwhelming, and the ensuing stress only worsened my symptoms. My mother and I found ourselves drowning in medical bills, unaware that my stepfather's employer had ceased paying our health insurance after his death. By the age of six, I was already receiving my first medical bills a burden far too heavy for a child to bear.

With no financial security and limited options, my mother made a difficult decision. Along with my newborn stepbrother, we moved to Sparta, Greece, to live with my aunt and uncle. What should have been a fresh start quickly turned into another period of turmoil. The drastic change in my environment, compounded by my untreated illness, led to a small nervous breakdown that lasted over a year. I was in constant pain, overwhelmed, and without access to proper medical care. Insurance was nonexistent, and there was no one to help me navigate my suffering.

After two years, we returned to the United States. My mother, determined to secure medical care for us, took a job in the healthcare industry. It was the only way she could obtain health insurance for our family, as no providers were willing to cover me due to my preexisting conditions. It was a cruel irony insurance companies, designed to help people in need, cared only about the financial risk I posed rather than my wellbeing.

With insurance in place, the medical appointments resumed. I was subjected to countless tests, procedures, and consultations. Gastrointestinal exams, colonoscopies, and biopsies became routine. It was an exhausting and invasive process, but finally, at the age of nine, I received the diagnosis that would shape the rest of my life I had Crohn's disease.

The diagnosis was a revelation and a heartbreak. On one hand, I finally had an explanation for the years of pain, but on the other, I realized that this wasn't something that could be easily cured. My family, like so many others, placed their trust in doctors, believing that every new medication or treatment was the key to managing my condition. But what we did not yet understand was that the food and medical industries operated in a cycle like a snake eating its own tail treating symptoms rather than addressing the root cause. We did not yet question the role of diet beyond avoiding certain foods, nor did we understand that the very treatments meant to help me could, in the long run, make living with Crohn's even more difficult.

Looking back, I can't help but think about how different my childhood might have been had I been diagnosed earlier and had we understood the deeper connection between food and health. Had we known to challenge the medical industry's one size fits all approach, perhaps the years of suffering could have been minimized. But life does not offer do overs it only offers lessons. And this was the first of many I would learn in my battle with Crohn's disease.

TEENS TO YOUNG ADULT LIFE

A Journey of Resilience: Living with

Crohn's Disease

From an early age, life posed challenges that most children never have to face, they were marked by an unrelenting struggle with Crohn's disease a chronic inflammatory bowel disease that causes inflammation of the digestive tract, leading to severe abdominal pain, diarrhea, fatigue, and malnutrition.

By the age of 11, a significant health scare led to a blood transfusion due to severe blood loss an event that would mark the beginning of a lifelong struggle with Crohn's disease. This early intervention triggered a cascade of medical treatments, dietary restrictions, and procedures aimed at controlling the symptoms and preventing complications.

The path through adolescence was riddled with countless attempts to manage Crohn's disease. Various diets were introduced, including elemental diets, anti-inflammatory plans, gluten free regimens, and even restrictive approaches like the carnivore diet. Alongside these dietary adjustments came a litany of medical procedures: colonoscopies, endoscopies, capsule endoscopies, CT scans, and countless blood tests, each providing pieces of the puzzle but never a complete solution. Medications such as cortisones, azathioprine, ciprofloxacin, and Asacol became routine, yet relief remained elusive.

At the age of 13, a significant surgical intervention marked a pivotal moment in my treatment journey. Initially under care at Lutheran General Hospital in Park Ridge (now part Advocate), I was transferred to Children's Memorial Hospital in Lincoln Park, Chicago (now known as Ann & Robert H. Lurie Children's Hospital), which was then recognized as a top-rated facility for pediatric gastrointestinal surgery. There, I underwent a bowel resection to remove a stricture in my small intestine. Despite the expertise involved and hopes for improvement, the complications from Crohn's persisted, continuing to challenge both my health and daily life. In the aftermath, I was placed on clear liquid diets, and at one point, I could not eat at all, relying instead on an IV PICC line for nutrition a stark reminder of the disease's toll on my body. Frequent absences from school, missing gym classes, and the inability to consume certain foods like milk, which triggered adverse reactions led to social isolation and even disciplinary issues, such as being reprimanded for refusing milk despite its detrimental effects. These experiences underscored the profound impact of the disease on both my personal life and education.

The years following this surgery brought additional burdens that deepened the strain. After my bowel resection, I lost my grandfather, a towering father figure in my life. A veteran of Greek war, he had immigrated to the United States in 1955 seeking opportunity, eventually raising three daughters, including my mother. His death, about a year after he insisted my mother enter her third marriage, left a void that echoed through our family. This third husband, an alcoholic, offered no stability or paternal presence for my brother or me; instead, his presence coupled with the grief of losing my grandfather piled stress atop an already fragile existence. The combination of chronic illness and a turbulent home life tested my resilience, yet it also fueled a longing for independence. By age 19, I seized the chance to move out, a step toward reclaiming control amid the chaos of disease and dysfunction.

Yet, amid these health battles, passions flourished. I feel music was my first real drug that made me feel good a lifeline that emerged at the age of five, when a deep love for it took root. This passion led to playing drums by nine and eventually stepping into the role of a DJ in my early teenage years. It expanded further into crafting custom music mixes and performing at events like weddings, bar mitzvahs, and school dances. Music became both an outlet and a source of joy, a steady rhythm cutting through the adversity of chronic illness.

The entrepreneurial spirit further extended into the world of car audio and custom car performance. Launching a venture called "Car Crazy," this passion quickly evolved into a successful business, with custom modified cars being shipped worldwide. Steve was building similar cars to the Fast and Furious movie before Fast and Furious was a movie or had been released. However, just as success was taking off, health complications returned with greater severity. By 17, frequent blood transfusions became necessary, and dietary changes intensified to manage internal bleeding more effectively.

At the age of 20, while many peers were celebrating milestones like their 21st birthdays, my life was defined by hospital stays and frequent blood transfusions. A persistent challenge during this time was the lack of clarity surrounding the cause of my chronic blood loss. Rather than investigating the root issue, medical professionals often attributed my symptoms to Crohn's disease without deeper exploration, leaving me with unanswered questions and ongoing uncertainty.

Transitioning from pediatric to adult care at the University of Chicago offered a glimmer of hope. I was referred to Dr. H, a physician widely regarded as a leading expert in Crohn's disease. Known for their involvement in advancing treatments and collaborating with pharmaceutical companies, Dr. H seemed poised to provide the specialized care I desperately needed. I entered this new phase of treatment with optimism, believing it could mark a turning point in my health journey.

Unfortunately, my experience with Dr. H fell short of expectations, and I came to view their care as Inadequate. Concerns arose about their approach, which at times felt dismissive and overly focused on standard protocols rather than addressing my individual needs. This experience was disheartening, particularly given Dr. H reputation. It led me to question the broader dynamics of medical care, including how certain physicians are elevated as experts without consistent accountability.

Reflecting on this, I've learned the importance of advocating for myself and seeking providers who prioritize thorough, patient centered care. While my journey with Crohn's disease remains complex, these experiences have underscored the need for a healthcare system that listens to patients and pursues root causes with diligence and compassion.

This journey is a testament to resilience and determination. Despite ongoing health challenges, the pursuit of passions and entrepreneurial dreams never wavered. From overcoming medical hurdles to achieving personal and professional milestones, this story reflects not just survival but the triumph of spirit against overwhelming odds.

YOUNG ADULT LIFE

Battling Shadows   Steve's Third Decade with Crohn's Disease

Steve's twenties were not adorned with the vibrant hues of youthful exuberance or the boundless freedom of carefree exploration. Instead, this decade unfurled as a relentless struggle not merely against the ravages of illness, but for dignity, comprehension, and the sheer will to endure.

The Ticking Clock: Early Trials and Surgical Ordeals

At the tender age of 25, when many of his contemporaries were scaling career heights or traversing distant lands, Steve stood at a harrowing crossroads. Another bowel resection loomed a procedure to excise the diseased segments of his intestine, marking his second such surgery. This invasive intervention, often a final bastion against the progression of Crohn's disease, carried the weight of potential complications. Entrusting his fate to Dr. H, a luminary in Crohn's treatment at the University of Chicago, Steve harbored fragile hope. Yet, the surgery yielded no respite, but a cascade of torment. Infections surged unchecked through his weakened frame, and fistulas aberrant passages linking intestine to skin or other organs erupted with merciless frequency. At his nadir, Steve bore the burden of approximately twelve active fistulas: half emerging from the surgical incision across his abdomen, the others tormenting his perianal region. Each fistula, an open wound, demanded ceaseless cleaning, packing, and draining as abscesses festered.

The aftermath of that second resection was a descent into sleepless agony. Emerging from the operating room, an unshakable premonition gripped him a visceral certainty that something had gone awry. He pleaded with his mother and those around him to extricate him from the hospital's grasp, a gut instinct he would never forget. For ten days, slumber eluded him entirely; no narcotic, sedative, or palliative could quell the war raging within. Dilaudid and methadone dulled the pain, but sleeping pills only deepened his discomfort. Stationed at the University of Chicago Hospital, Steve oscillated in and out of its sterile halls for over two years, with one grueling stretch spanning seven months. His mother and girlfriend stood as unwavering sentinels by his side, yet even their devotion could not coax his eyes to close. Nights blurred into a vigil with nurses, whom he pressed to decipher his charts finding in their compassion a solace often absent from physicians. Scans CT, MRI, fistulograms numbered in the dozens, orchestrated by specialists wielding dyes and machines, while mornings greeted him with X-rays from his bed. Weakness consumed him, yet an indomitable will drove him to rise.

By the eighth day, frustration morphed into a barrage of questions queries so piercing that his surgeon, Dr. F ceased to reappear. Steve conjectured darkly: had the surgeon been unfit, or had an intern's unsteady hand botched the procedure under inadequate oversight? This suspicion, perhaps a conspiracy born of desperation, lingered unresolved. As the ordeal intensified, Steve found himself on what felt like a deathbed severely malnourished, his organs beginning to shut down from sepsis. The brink of collapse loomed, a stark testament to the toll of the surgery's aftermath, yet his resolve held firm, a flicker of defiance amid the encroaching darkness.

The Pharmaceutical Maze: Immunosuppressants and Shattered Promises

In a bid to stem the tide of infection, fistulas, and inflammation, Steve's physicians turned to a formidable arsenal of immunosuppressive biologics: Remicade and then Humira. These agents, engineered to temper the immune system's fervor, promised relief but delivered a labyrinth of disillusionment.

• Remicade (Infliximab): Administered intravenously in a hospital setting, this biologic a fusion of rat protein and human TNF inhibitors was pioneered in the late 1990s for Crohn's patients unresponsive to conventional therapies. Prescribed to Steve under Dr. H's care, it aimed to neutralize inflammation. Yet, its side effects ranging from infusion reactions to heightened infection risk compounded his woes, and its efficacy waned as his body rebelled.

• Humira (Adalimumab): For a decade, this self injected treatment arrived at Steve's doorstep, a subcutaneous lifeline approved in 2002 for Crohn's management. Targeting TNFalpha, it sought to quell inflammation at home. But prolonged use birthed antibodies, rendering it impotent, a resistance confirmed years later by a Pythagoras Humira antibody test Steve demanded after his pleas were long ignored.

• Entyvio (Vedolizumab): Introduced later in Steve's journey, this 2014approved biologic offered a novel approach, selectively blocking gut specific inflammation via integrin inhibition. Administered via infusion, it promised fewer systemic side effects but faltered against Steve's relentless disease, leaving him grasping for alternatives.

• Cimzia (Certolizumab Pegol): Another injectable, approved in 2008, this TNF blocker aimed to suppress immune overactivity with a pegylated structure for prolonged action. For Steve, it joined the chorus of false hopes, its benefits eclipsed by his body's growing defiance.

These cutting-edge therapies, heralded as medical marvels, unraveled a grim truth: Steve's immune system turned traitor, forging antibodies against the very drugs meant to save him. Infusions and injections became rituals of futility; his concerns brushed aside until the antibody test laid bare a decade of misplaced trust in Humira.

The Crohn's Conspiracy: Medicine as Commerce

Through this odyssey, Steve glimpsed what he termed the "Crohn's Conspiracy" not a clandestine cabal, but a stark indictment of healthcare's systemic flaws. Expensive biologics flowed freely, their costs rubber-stamped by insurers despite evident failure. His intuition, urging antibody testing, was dismissed, underscoring a troubling silence around patient voices. Studies hinting at risks like cancer tied to drugs like Humira and Remicade fueled his suspicion: was profit, not healing, the true north of this pharmaceutical compass?

Finding Sanctuary: Cannabis as Salvation

Amid the wreckage of conventional medicine, Steve stumbled upon an unlikely redeemer: cannabis. Initially dubious, he embraced it at 26, on what felt like his deathbed at the University of Chicago. Friends and family, crowding his hospital room during monthslong stays, shared the plant in his darkest hours. Its effects easing nausea, quelling spasms, restoring appetite, and granting rest unlocked a revelation. Unlike biologics, cannabis offered clarity, fueling his research into its anti-inflammatory and analgesic virtues. Though illegal and taboo in medical circles then, it became his lifeline, lifting him from that bed and the hospital's grip. Far from a gateway drug, cannabis severed his reliance on opioids prescribed narcotics that once tethered him to addiction's edge. To Steve, it was no mere intoxicant but a vegetable, akin to ancient amaranth, a natural ally in his fight.

The Silent Exile of Chronic Illness

Beyond physical torment, Steve's twenties bore the weight of profound isolation. Crohn's, an invisible scourge, cloaked its brutality from the world. Months in hospitals, punctuated by invasive procedures, distanced him from life's rhythm. Friendships frayed, romances crumbled, and career dreams faded all sacrificed to the altar of survival.

A Redefined Valor

By his twenties' end, Steve transcended mere endurance. He emerged an advocate, wielding research, skepticism of medical dogma, and alternative therapies as his arsenal. This decade forged not just his bond with Crohn's, but a new paradigm of living with chronic illness resilient, inquisitive, and defiant in a world blind to invisible suffering.

ADULT LIFE & EPIPHANY

The Crohn's Conspiracy – Steve's Third Decade

The third decade of Steve's existence was not a mere extension of his skirmish with Crohn's disease. It unfurled as a profound immersion into research, advocacy, and unorthodox experimentation a period illuminated by scientific fervor, dogged perseverance, and a burgeoning suspicion that the medical establishment's failures were not aberrations, but threads in a systemic tapestry of neglect. This era saw Steve's struggle transcend personal endurance, evolving into a bold challenge against the entrenched narrative of Crohn's and a quest to master his own affliction.

A New Scientific Obsession: The Cannabis Revelation

By his thirties, Steve's faith in conventional medicine had eroded to a husk. Years of biologics Remicade, Humira, Entyvio delivered not healing or insight into root causes, but a litany of side effects and unfulfilled promises. Battered by these pharmaceutical titans, he turned to an unlikely savior: cannabis. Long scorned by medical orthodoxy, it granted what costly infusions and injections could not genuine relief. Beyond mere pain suppression, cannabis restored a semblance of life's richness, soothing nausea, calming spasms, and luring sleep where none had dared linger.

This awakening sparked a fascination with cannabinoids, the plant's potent compounds, with CBD (cannabidiol) shining as a beacon for its non-psychoactive, anti inflammatory prowess. In 2010, this pursuit propelled him to California, chasing CBD's untapped potential. His journey soon veered to Colorado, a vanguard of medicinal cannabis innovation, where he sought the Stanley Brothers of Realm of Caring, creators of Charlotte's Web. That initial 2010 meeting disappointed empty assurances drowned in hype but it galvanized him to forge his own path. Colorado, with medical cannabis legalized in 2000 via Amendment 20 and recreational use sanctioned in 2012 through Amendment 64, pulsed with opportunity. By January 1, 2014, licensed dispensaries thrived, and Steve immersed himself in this ecosystem, collaborating with growers, extractors, and breeders cultivating plants rich in targeted cannabinoids.

Farmers presented CBD in diverse forms tinctures, oils, edibles but Steve's body rebelled against their common carriers: MCT coconut oil, alcohol, glycerin, and seed oils. From this resistance emerged a groundbreaking innovation: an extra virgin olive oil infused with full spectrum cannabinoids. Sourced from his family's Olive groves in Greece and blended with organically grown Colorado cannabis, this farm to table tincture married the plant's therapeutic power with olive oil's unadulterated purity. Bioliveit Cannabinoids was started in 2015, it stood as a bespoke triumph tailored to his unique needs, offering not just symptom relief but a bold reclamation of agency.

Steve turned to cannabis, finding solace in Cannabis Cannabinoids with CBD Cannabidiol being just one of the over 100 discovered Cannabinoids in the cannabis plant. Where the medical establishment settled for fleeting fixes, Steve crafted a lasting remedy, a testament to his defiance and ingenuity.

The Crohn's Conspiracy: A Hidden Bacterial Culprit

Steve's inquiry pressed beyond cannabis, plunging into contentious terrain: the theory that Crohn's might not be solely autoimmune, but rooted in bacterial treachery. At its core lay MAP Mycobacterium avium subspecies paratuberculosis a stealthy kind to tuberculosis and leprosy. Mainstream medicine largely scoffed, yet a rising chorus of international studies fingered MAP as Crohn's shadowy provocateur.

This bacterium, mutated from tuberculosis into paratuberculosis through antibacterial resistance, had shed its cell wall. Standard tests, reliant on dyeing cellular walls for microscopic scrutiny, failed against this wraith, leaving MAP undetected and untreated. Steve unearthed a damning contradiction: doctors wielded immunosuppressants Remicade, Humira, Cimzia to douse inflammation, blind to evidence that this blaze was the body's retort to MAP's parasitic siege. These drugs, he argued, crippled the immune system's natural defense, misdiagnosing a valiant response as an overactive flaw. Remicade's label warned of tuberculosis outbreaks; Humira and Cimzia bore cancer risks Steve knew peers stricken within a year. Each new immunosuppressant triggered a tuberculosis test, a bitter irony as these treatments fueled the infections they claimed to quell.

This mistreatment spiraled patients into agony intensifying pain, futile surgeries, barbaric eviscerations, and bowel resections that scarred lives irrevocably. Millions endured this torment, a reality Steve refused to ignore. He forged ties with global pioneers like Thomas Borody, an Australian gastroenterologist who devised triple antibiotic therapy: Rifampin (a tuberculosis bulwark), Clarithromycin (a broad-spectrum sentinel), and Clofazimine (a leprosy remedy with anti-inflammatory might). Before embracing this, Steve made one final pilgrimage to the University of Chicago in 2018, clutching a decade's research. Seeking Dr. R, then the Crohn's luminary at this top-rated institution, he hoped for dialogue on antiMAP treatment. Instead, he met gaslighting anew documented in emails he'd eagerly share. Dr. R dismissed his pleas, concocted a fictitious diagnosis, and flared Steve's condition, leaving him bedridden. When Steve rallied to confront him via email, Dr. R dodged, claiming antiMAP therapy suited only those post bowel removal with ostomy bags a refrain echoing his youth. Promises of stem cell fistula treatments dissolved into legal excuses, a farce Dr. R later glossed over in a UChicago Medicine article, musing that Crohn's might span 50 to 100 overlapping diseases yet offering no clarity.

Undeterred, Steve pursued the triple antibiotic regimen for two and a half years, clinging to hope it might strike Crohn's root and ease his fistulas and infections. The results tantalized relief flickered until systemic roadblocks, like insurance intransigence, dimmed the flame. Over 26 years, he'd poured over $500,000 into Blue Cross Blue Shield via premiums and deductibles a king's ransom for a system that repaid him with inertia.

A Decade of Defiance

This third decade forged Steve into more than a survivor it cast him as a relentless seeker, challenging medical dogma with cannabis and antiMAP (Mycobacterium avium subspecies paratuberculosis) theories, and wresting control from a faltering establishment. Yet, this period was also defined by an unrelenting struggle against a singular, life altering recommendation: an ostomy bag. From ages 26 to 37, Steve faced a barrage of pressure from at least 20 doctors across hospitals and university clinics, each insisting that an ostomy was his only viable option. Time and again, he was urged to defer to his primary physician, hailed as the expert, despite his instincts screaming otherwise.

Young and resolute, Steve refused to accept a bag hanging from his body as his fate. Beyond the visceral aversion, he harbored a deep mistrust of surgeons, fearing their interventions would inflict further damage and expose him to a cascade of infections a risk he couldn't bear to imagine, given the fragility Crohn's had already imposed. For over a decade, he fought back, rejecting the chorus of medical consensus with a tenacity born of necessity and defiance. This was no mere act of rebellion; it was a calculated stand against a system that too often seemed resigned to managing symptoms rather than seeking solutions.

Through this grueling battle, Steve's fight evolved beyond mere survival. It became a quest for truth a beacon for the millions ensnared in Crohn's silent conspiracy. Armed with alternative approaches and an unyielding will, he carved out a path that defied the odds, proving that resilience and skepticism could illuminate a way forward where conventional medicine had faltered.

MYCOBACTERIUM AVIUM PARATUBERCULOSIS:

Pioneers Koch, Johne, and Frothingham

In the shadowy annals of medical history, Mycobacterium avium paratuberculosis (MAP) emerges as a elusive pathogen, long associated with chronic intestinal disease in animals and increasingly implicated in human Crohns disease. This bacterium, resilient and insidious, has sparked debates that echo through time, from the laboratories of 19th-century pioneers to today's contentious research. This chapter spotlights three key figures: Robert Koch, whose postulates set the gold standard for proving infectious causation; Heinrich Hermann Albert Johne, the German pathologist who first described paratuberculosis in cattle; and Langdon Frothingham, his American collaborator who helped isolate the culprit. Their work laid the foundation for understanding MAP, yet it also highlights the frustrations in linking it to Crohn's, a disease that defies easy classification. As a Crohn's patient whose journey has been marked by revelations about potential infectious triggers, I see their legacies as both inspirational and cautionary. In a world where Crohn's is often dismissed as purely autoimmune, costing patients $10,000 to $30,000 annually in treatments that manage but rarely cure, revisiting these scientists reveals a conspiracy of sorts: a reluctance to embrace infectious models that could upend profitable paradigms. Through their stories, we uncover MAPs history, its veterinary roots, and its controversial leap to human health, demanding we question why such foundational work remains on the fringes.

Robert Koch: The Architect of Infectious Proof

Robert Koch (1843-1910), the German physician and microbiologist, revolutionized medicine with his rigorous approach to identifying disease-causing microbes. Born in Clausthal, Koch studied medicine at the University of Gottingen and later worked as a district medical officer. His breakthrough came in 1876 when he isolated Bacillus anthracis, the cause of anthrax, using innovative techniques like potato slices for culturing. This paved the way for his famous postulates, outlined in 1890: (1) the microorganism must be found in abundance in all organisms suffering from the disease, but not in healthy ones; (2) it must be isolated from a diseased organism and grown in pure culture; (3) the cultured microorganism should cause disease when introduced into a healthy organism; and (4) it must be re-isolated from the inoculated, diseased host and identified as identical to the original.

Kochs postulates became the cornerstone of infectious disease research, earning him the 1905 Nobel Prize in Physiology or Medicine for his work on tuberculosis. He isolated Mycobacterium tuberculosis in 1882, developing staining methods that revealed acid-fast bacilli, a characteristic shared by MAP. His emphasis on pure cultures and animal models transformed vague associations into proven causations, influencing generations of scientists.

Yet, Kochs legacy casts a long shadow over MAP and Crohn's. MAP, a slow-growing mycobacterium, is notoriously difficult to culture, often requiring months or specialized media. In Crohn's patients, MAP is detected in varying frequencies, from 50% to 92% in some studies, but not universally, violating Kochs first postulate. Ethical barriers prevent fulfilling the third: inoculating humans, especially children where Crohn's often begins, is unthinkable. As microbiologist Michael Collins noted, direct evidence for MAP causing Crohn's is impossible due to these constraints. This rigidity has allowed skeptics to dismiss the MAP-Crohn's link, favoring autoimmune theories that sustain billion-dollar biologic markets.

For me, Kochs postulates represent both genius and limitation. In my young adult years I accepted the autoimmune label, but learning of MAP challenged that. Kochs framework, while brilliant for acute infections, falters for chronic, stealthy pathogens like MAP, highlighting how outdated standards can obscure truths.

Heinrich Hermann Albert Johne: Uncovering the Bovine Scourge

Heinrich Hermann Albert Johne (1839-1910), a German veterinary pathologist, is indelibly linked to MAP through his discovery of paratuberculosis, or Johne's disease. Born in Dresden, Johne trained at the Veterinary School in Dresden and later became a professor of pathology there. His work focused on animal diseases, particularly those affecting livestock, in an era when agriculture was vital to economies.

In 1895, Johne examined a cow from Saxony suffering from chronic diarrhea and wasting, symptoms unresponsive to tuberculosis treatments. Microscopic analysis revealed thickened intestinal walls riddled with acid-fast bacilli, resembling avian tuberculosis but distinct from bovine TB. Johne hypothesized an infectious cause, publishing his findings in the Deutsche Zeitschrift fur Tiermedizin und Vergleichende Pathologie. He described the disease as a pseudotuberculous enteritis, noting granulomatous lesions similar to those in Crohn's.

Johnes collaboration with American veterinarian Langdon Frothingham, detailed below, confirmed the bacillus as unique. They concluded it was avian TB adapted to cattle, though later classifications identified it as Mycobacterium avium subsp. paratuberculosis. Johne's disease, named after him, spreads via fecal-oral routes, contaminating pastures and milk, with infected animals shedding billions of bacteria.

Johne's work was groundbreaking, alerting farmers to a costly scourge: infected herds suffer reduced milk production and early culling, costing the U.S. dairy industry $200-250 million annually. His staining techniques and pathological descriptions advanced mycobacteriology, influencing human medicine.

The leap to Crohn's came later. In 1913, Scottish surgeon Thomas Kennedy Dalziel noted similarities between Johnes and human intestinal TB, now recognized as Crohn's-like. Modern studies detect MAP in Crohn's tissues, with genetic susceptibilities like NOD2 mutations impairing macrophage responses to mycobacteria. Johne's legacy thus fuels the MAP-Crohn's hypothesis, suggesting zoonotic transmission via dairy or water.

As a patient, Johne's discovery resonates deeply. Learning MAP survives pasteurization explained my dairy-triggered flares. His veterinary focus underscores a missed opportunity: if animal health warranted such scrutiny, why not human?

Langdon Frothingham: Bridging Continents and Confirming the Pathogen

Langdon Frothingham (1867-1935), an American veterinarian and pathologist, played a pivotal role in confirming Johne's findings and isolating MAP. Born in Boston, Frothingham studied at Harvard Veterinary School and later worked at the U.S. Bureau of Animal Industry. His expertise in tuberculosis led to collaborations across borders.

In 1895, Frothingham received samples from Johne and independently analyzed them. His examinations corroborated the presence of acid-fast bacilli in the cows intestines, ruling out standard TB strains. Their joint publication solidified paratuberculosis as a distinct entity. Frothingham went further, attempting cultures and animal inoculations to fulfill emerging standards like Kochs postulates.

By 1909, Frothingham successfully isolated the bacterium from U.S. cattle, proving its presence beyond Europe. His work at the Massachusetts Agricultural Experiment Station advanced diagnostics, including the johnin skin test, analogous to the tuberculin test. Frothingham emphasized control measures: culling infected animals and hygiene to prevent spread.

Frothinghams contributions extended MAPs recognition in North America, influencing policies that mitigated economic losses. His emphasis on chronic, subclinical infections mirrored Crohn's relapsing nature.

In the Crohn's context, Frothinghams isolations provided strains for modern research. Studies using these have shown MAPs viability in pasteurized milk (up to 18% of samples) and its detection in Crohn's patients blood and tissues. His work supports theories of environmental exposure, with MAP contaminating water supplies and surviving chlorination.

Frothinghams transatlantic collaboration highlights sciences global nature, yet it contrasts with todays siloed research. For me, his persistence in isolating a tricky pathogen inspires hope for Crohn's breakthroughs, despite systemic resistance.

Linking the Pioneers: MAPs Path from Veterinary to Human Disease

Koch, Johne, and Frothingham form a triad in MAPs history. Kochs postulates provided the framework Johne and Frothingham used to characterize paratuberculosis. Their descriptions of granulomatous enteritis in cattle eerily parallel Crohn's, first detailed by Burrill Crohn in 1932.

The connection strengthened in the 1980s when Rod Chiodini isolated MAP from Crohn's tissues, echoing Johne and Frothinghams methods. Debates rage: MAP meets some postulates in animals but falters in humans due to ethics and variability. Critics cite inconsistent detection, yet advocates point to improved PCR and culture techniques showing higher prevalence.

This history exposes barriers: veterinary-human divides, funding biases toward autoimmune models, and agribusiness reluctance to acknowledge zoonotic risks. The $13 billion Crohn's market favors biologics like Humira ($20 billion peak) over antibiotics targeting MAP, which could cost $1,000 to $2,000 per course.

Personal Reflections: Echoes of History in My Struggle

Reflecting on these pioneers, I see parallels to my journey. Kochs rigor inspired my quest for proof; Johne's descriptions matched my symptoms; Frothinghams isolations validated my suspicions. Yet, the failure to fully apply their lessons to Crohn's fuels frustration. Why, in 2025, do guidelines ignore MAP while patients suffer? Their work demands we bridge gaps, funding zoonotic research and challenging dogmas.

Mycobacterium avium paratuberculosis, through the lenses of Koch, Johne, and Frothingham, reveals a pathogen with deep roots and profound implications. Kochs postulates set standards; Johne and Frothingham uncovered its veterinary toll. Their legacies urge us to confront MAPs role in Crohn's, dismantling conspiracies of inaction. As patients, we stand unbowed, unbroken, invoking their spirit to demand cures over complacency.

REDHILL BIOPHARMA:
Pioneers in MAP Research Amid Global Inertia

In the complex landscape of Crohn's disease research, RedHill Biopharma stands out as a bold leader in pursuing treatments targeting Mycobacterium avium subspecies paratuberculosis (MAP). This Israeli-based company has advanced therapies like RHB-104 and RHB-204, securing patents and conducting groundbreaking studies that challenge the autoimmune dogma. But why is RedHill allowed to forge ahead while major players in the USA and UK seem stagnant? How does Israel facilitate such progress when others lag? This chapter explores these questions, uncovering the regulatory, economic, and systemic barriers that stifle MAP research elsewhere. Drawing from RedHills patent portfolio, clinical trials, and the broader Crohn's landscape, we will examine the conspiracy of silence: a profit-driven system that favors expensive biologics over potentially curative antibiotics. As a Crohn's patient who has studied suppressed research, I see RedHills efforts as a glimmer of hope but also a stark indictment of global inequities in medical innovation. In a world where Crohn's costs patients $10,000 to $30,000 annually and the market swells to $13 billion, RedHills path raises uncomfortable truths about who controls the cure.

RedHill Biopharma: Origins and Focus on MAP

RedHill Biopharma, founded in 2009 and headquartered in Tel Aviv, Israel, with a U.S. subsidiary in Raleigh, North Carolina, specializes in gastrointestinal and infectious diseases. Their entry into Crohn's research began in 2010 with the acquisition of rights to a novel antibiotic combination from the University of Central Florida, evolving into

RHB-104, a fixed-dose capsule of clarithromycin, rifabutin, and clofazimine designed to eradicate MAP. This therapy builds on the hypothesis that MAP, linked to Johne's disease in cattle, triggers Crohn's in susceptible humans.

RedHills commitment is evident in their robust patent portfolio. They hold multiple U.S. patents for RHB-104s formulation and use in Crohn's, including allowances in 2018 and 2016 that extend protection to 2041. These patents cover the drugs composition, methods of treatment, and diagnostic integrations, ensuring exclusivity. RHB-204, an optimized successor with a reduced pill burden, inherits this intellectual property, positioning RedHill as a leader in anti-MAP therapy.

Their ability to secure patents stems from standard pharmaceutical practices: innovation, filing via bodies like the USPTO, and compliance with international treaties. RedHills dual Israeli-U.S. presence facilitates global filings, leveraging Israels strong intellectual property laws, which align with TRIPS agreements. This setup allows them to own and develop MAP patents without unique permission; it is business as usual for a biopharma firm investing in research and development.

Groundbreaking Studies: From RHB-104 to RHB-204
RedHills clinical trials underscore their pioneering role. The MAP US Phase 3 study, a randomized, double-blind trial with 331 U.S. patients, met its primary endpoint in 2019: 36.7% remission at week 26 versus 22.4% placebo (p=0.0048). Full results, published in

2024 in Antibiotics, confirmed 64% increased efficacy and endoscopic improvements. An open-label extension further supported durability.

Building on this, RedHill advanced RHB-204. In July 2025, the FDA provided positive feedback for a Phase 2 study, the first in MAP-positive Crohn's patients, focusing on mucosal remission and MAP eradication. This innovative trial, planned for 2025, highlights RedHills agility in navigating U.S. regulations.

RedHill conducts studies internationally, including in Australia and New Zealand. Their Israeli base does not restrict them; rather25% pill burden improves compliance, and partnerships bolster funding. Israels vibrant biotech ecosystem, with government incentives like R&D grants from the Israel Innovation Authority, supports such ventures.

Why Limited MAP Research in the USA and UK?

Despite RedHills U.S. trials, broader MAP research in the USA and UK remains limited, fueling questions of suppression. The MAP hypothesis is controversial: while evidence mounts, with MAP detected in up to 92% of Crohn's tissues, critics argue inconsistent findings and failure to meet Kochs postulates due to ethical constraints. No agency, like the CDC or USDA, declares MAP zoonotic, citing only indirect evidence.

Funding shortages plague the field. Pharmaceutical giants prioritize biologics, such as Humira, which peaked at $20 billion, shunning cheap antibiotics that could disrupt markets. In the USA, NIH grants favor autoimmune models; MAP studies receive scant support. The UK has explored an anti-MAP vaccine in a 2018-2019 trial, but results were preliminary, with no large-scale follow-up.

Interdisciplinary barriers hinder progress: gastroenterologists dominate, sidelining microbiologists and veterinarians. Regulatory caution, with concerns about long-term antibiotic resistance, slows approvals. Economic ties to agribusiness, wary of MAP in dairy implications, add pressure.

This inertia contrasts with RedHills investor-backed model, allowing them to pursue MAP despite mainstream skepticism.

Israels Edge: Innovation Hub in a Global Landscape

Israels allowance for such studies is not exclusive; RedHill operates globally. However, Israels ecosystem fosters biotech innovation. Dubbed the Start-Up Nation, it boasts high R&D spending (5% of GDP), tax incentives, and a dense network of universities and incubators. RedHill benefits from this, securing patents and partnerships efficiently.

Unlike the USA or UK, where big pharma dominates and MAP is marginalized, Israels nimble firms like RedHill can pivot to niche areas. No unique permission exists; trials follow international guidelines, but Israels regulatory body, the Ministry of Health, is agile, facilitating early-stage work. RedHills treatments are not exclusively available in Israel; they are in development for global markets, with U.S. FDA engagement.

This disparity highlights a conspiracy: entrenched interests in larger economies suppress disruptive therapies, while smaller nations innovate freely.

Personal Reflections: A Patients View on Global Disparities

Reflecting on my Crohn's journey, RedHills progress is bittersweet. I detailed my epiphany questioning autoimmune narratives; MAP research validated that. Yet, living in a system where U.S. and UK research lags, I have faced barriers to anti-MAP trials. Why must an Israeli company lead while patients elsewhere wait? It is a stark reminder of profit over people; the $35 billion IBD market by 2034 depends on chronicity. RedHills patents offer hope, but global inertia fuels my advocacy for equitable research.

RedHill Biopharmas ability to run MAP studies and own patents stems from innovation, compliance, and Israels supportive ecosystem, not exclusive privileges. Limited progress in the USA and UK arises from controversy, funding biases, and economic motives that favor biologics over cures. Israels edge lies in agility, not isolation; yet this global disparity exposes the Crohn's Conspiracy: a system where breakthroughs are siloed, leaving patients unbowed but unbroken, demanding universal access to truth and treatment.

CROHN'S DISEASE AS A PROFIT MACHINE
MACHINE
The Economic Conspiracy

In the shadowed corridors of modern medicine, where hope is peddled in pill form and remission is a fleeting promise, Crohn's disease stands as a testament to the commodification of suffering. For decades, I've navigated the treacherous waters of this chronic illness, witnessing firsthand how a potentially curable condition has been transformed into a perpetual revenue stream for pharmaceutical giants. This chapter peels back the layers of what I call the "Crohn's Conspiracy" a systemic entanglement where profit motives eclipse patient cures. Drawing from the groundbreaking work on MAP (Mycobacterium avium subspecies paratuberculosis) explored in previous chapters, we'll examine how the industry perpetuates lifelong dependency through expensive biologics and immunosuppressants, while sidelining affordable alternatives like antibiotics. The numbers are staggering: a global market worth billions, individual patient costs soaring into the tens of thousands annually, and a deliberate resistance to paradigms that could end the cycle. As someone who's felt the financial sting alongside the physical pain, I argue that Crohn's isn't just a disease it's a business model designed to keep us hooked, hopeful, and perpetually paying.

The Historical Roots of Profitable Management

Crohn's disease, first described in 1932 by Dr. Burrill B. Crohn and colleagues, has evolved from a mysterious ailment to a well orchestrated profit center. In the early days, treatments were rudimentary: surgeries to resect inflamed bowel sections, corticosteroids to tamp down inflammation, and a resigned acceptance that relapse was inevitable. But as medical science advanced, so did the opportunities for monetization. The shift from viewing Crohn's as a possible infectious disease potentially linked to pathogens like MAP to an autoimmune disorder requiring ongoing immunosuppression was pivotal. This reclassification wasn't merely scientific; it aligned perfectly with the pharmaceutical industry's strengths in developing high margin, patent protected drugs.

By the 1990s, the introduction of biologics like infliximab (Remicade) and adalimumab (Humira) marked a turning point. These drugs, engineered to block inflammatory pathways, offered symptom relief but no cure. Why pursue eradication when management ensures repeat customers? Historical analyses, such as those from the 1990s, hypothesized that a drug reducing non drug medical costs by 20% while doubling drug expenses could still lower overall costs. Yet, the reality diverged: biologics ballooned expenses without altering the disease's chronic nature. This era solidified Crohn's as a "lifelong condition," a phrase that echoes in doctor's offices and pharmaceutical boardrooms alike, translating to sustained revenue.

The economic framework was set: diagnose early, prescribe indefinitely, and profit handsomely. As global awareness grew, so did the market. Today, the Crohn's disease treatment sector is valued at over $13 billion, projected to reach $17.4 billion by 2033, growing at a compound annual rate of 6.4%. North America alone accounts for billions, with the U.S. inflammatory bowel disease (IBD) market hitting $11.85 billion in 2023. These figures aren't abstract they represent the monetization of misery, where each flare up feeds the machine.

The Pharmaceutical Goldmine: Billions in Biologics

At the heart of this conspiracy lies the biologics bonanza. Drugs like Humira and Remicade aren't just treatments; they're cash cows. Humira, AbbVie's blockbuster, generated over $20 billion in annual sales at its peak, much of it from IBD indications including Crohn's. Remicade, from Janssen, follows suit with billions in revenue. These monoclonal antibodies target tumor necrosis factor (TNF), quelling inflammation but requiring regular infusions or injections often for life.

The costs are exorbitant. A single vial of Remicade can run $987, with regimens demanding multiple vials per infusion, pushing annual expenses to $20,000 $40,000. Humira's list price can exceed $85,000 yearly without insurance, though biosimilars have introduced some competition, dropping prices to around $12,000 for generics. Even with insurance, out of pocket costs average $606 annually for medications alone, per patient surveys. For those on biologics, the burden multiplies: one study pegged yearly costs at over $57,000 for combination therapies.

Why so pricey? Patents protect these drugs for decades, stifling competition. Marketing budgets swell to influence prescribers think lavish dinners, sponsored conferences, and direct to consumer ads that normalize lifelong dependency. The inflammatory bowel disease treatment market, encompassing

Crohn's and ulcerative colitis, is forecasted to hit $35.88 billion by 2034, driven by these high-cost therapies. Pharmaceutical executives tout innovation, but the reality is a model where R&D costs are recouped manifold through inflated pricing, often subsidized by taxpayers via insurance premiums and government programs.

Contrast this with potential cures. As discussed in chapters on Rod Chiodini and RedHill Biopharma, anti-MAP therapies like RHB 104 use off patent antibiotics clarithromycin, rifabutin, clofazimine costing pennies compared to biologics. Phase 3 trials showed 64% increased efficacy in remission rates, yet adoption lags. Why? A cure disrupts the profit pipeline. If MAP eradication proved viable for a subset of patients, billions in biologic sales could evaporate. The industry's resistance isn't overt but insidious: underfunding MAP research, emphasizing autoimmune models in guidelines, and prioritizing symptom suppressing drugs in pipelines.

Lifelong Dependency: The Cycle of Costs and Control

Crohn's is framed as incurable, ensuring patients remain in the system indefinitely. Diagnosis often hits in one's 20s, prime earning years, yet the disease extracts a toll: average annual care costs hit $30,000 in the first year, stabilizing at $10,000 $12,000 thereafter. This includes not just drugs but hospitalizations (up to 20% of patients annually), surgeries (30 55% within 10 years), and ER visits.

Indirect costs amplify the burden. Missed work averages 9 days yearly for Crohn's patients versus 5 for healthy individuals, translating to hundreds in lost wages. Productivity dips, with 43% reporting inability to perform daily tasks during flares. Mental health suffers too twice the anxiety and depression rates adding therapy costs of $100 $200 per session.

The economic impact is profound. A 2019 Crohn's & Colitis Foundation study highlighted $30,000 initial year expenses, with biologics driving disparities: users incur 2-3 times higher costs. Globally, IBD costs society billions in lost productivity and healthcare. In the U.S., 23% face financial hardships from medical bills, 16% skip doses due to cost.

This dependency isn't accidental. Guidelines emphasize escalation to biologics after milder therapies fail, creating a funnel to high profit drugs. Maintenance regimens infusions every 8 weeks lock in revenue. Even when remission is achieved, discontinuation risks relapse, perpetuating the cycle. Bowel rest or nutritional therapies, cheaper alternatives, are sidelined in favor of pharmaceutical interventions.

Suppression of Alternatives: The MAP Hypothesis Under Siege

The MAP hypothesis, positing Crohn's as an infectious disease treatable with antibiotics, threatens this empire. Pioneers like Chiodini isolated MAP in Crohn's tissues in the 1980s, with studies detecting it in up to 92% of patients. Animal models confirm causation, and small trials show remission rates surpassing standards.

Yet, resistance persists. Critics cite inconsistent detection, but this masks deeper motives. Large scale MAP studies receive scant funding; pharmaceutical grants favor biologics. RedHill's RHB 104, despite positive Phase 3 data (36.7% remission vs. 22.4% placebo), faces regulatory hurdles. The 2025 FDA feedback on successor RHB 204 is promising, but slow progress highlights inertia.

Why the drag? A cure via cheap antibiotics potentially $1,000 $2,000 per course undermines the $12 billion Crohn's market. Public health implications, like MAP in dairy, could disrupt agribusiness allies. Instead, the narrative clings to autoimmunity, where suppression, not eradication, reigns. Articles lament "held hostage" cures, echoing my sentiment: promising anti MAP therapies succeed individually but fail systemically due to profit priorities.

The Patient Burden: Stories from the Frontlines
As a Crohn's warrior, I've tallied the toll. Early years meant steroids and immunosuppressants, affordable but side effect laden. Epiphany struck with MAP research switching to plant based diets, avoiding potential sources, and seeking antibiotic trials. Yet, access barriers persist: doctors dismissive, insurers favoring biologics.

Surveys mirror this: 35% see providers 1-2 times yearly, 37% 3 4, 21% 5+. Each visit chips away at savings. Emergency flares add hundreds; surgeries, thousands. Mentally, the grind erodes therapy essential but costly.

Community voices amplify: forums buzz with biosimilar hopes, yet many forego care due to expense. The conspiracy isn't faceless; it's in denied claims, inflated bills, and deferred dreams.

Personal Reflections: From Victim to Advocate
Reflecting on my journey from childhood diagnosis to adult advocacy I've seen the machine's gears. I chronicled personal epochs; here, the economic veil lifts. MAP insights offered hope, but systemic blocks fueled rage. I've advocated for reform: funding MAP trials, capping drug prices, prioritizing cures.

This isn't paranoia; it's pattern recognition. Bayer's legacy hints at corporate sins; extend to today's titans. Profit over people? Unacceptable.

Crohn's as a profit disease isn't hyperbole it's harsh reality. Billions flow while patients pay dearly. Yet, cracks appear: biosimilars erode monopolies, RedHill advances, awareness grows. We must demand transparency, fund alternatives, and unite; unbowed, unbroken. But now, empowered to dismantle the machine.

HIDDEN TREATMENTS AND ERASED DATA
The Suppression of Crohn's Cures

In the shadowed corners of medical research, where breakthroughs are celebrated and failures buried, Crohn's disease stands as a stark example of how potential cures can be sidelined for profit. For decades, I have battled the invisible chains of this illness, only to uncover that promising treatments, rooted in the infectious origins of Crohn's, have been systematically downplayed, their data twisted or ignored. This chapter exposes the Crohn's Conspiracy at its most insidious: the deliberate suppression of the Mycobacterium avium paratuberculosis (MAP) hypothesis and related therapies. Drawing on reanalyzed trials, overlooked studies, and the stark contrast between cheap antibiotics and billion dollar biologics, we will explore how pharmaceutical interests, regulatory inertia, and flawed research designs have hidden paths to remission or cure. As a patient who has felt the weight of these omissions, I present proof from published evidence, demanding we question why effective treatments remain obscured while suffering persists.

The MAP Hypothesis: A Century of Suppression

The idea that Crohn's disease might stem from an infectious agent like MAP is not new; it dates back over a century. In 1913, TK Dalziel noted striking similarities between Crohn's and Johnes disease in cattle, a chronic enteritis caused by MAP. Yet, despite these parallels, the MAP hypothesis has been relegated to the fringes of medical discourse. Why? The answer lies in a web of scientific, ethical, and economic barriers that amount to suppression.

MAP, a resilient bacterium that survives pasteurization and contaminates dairy and water, has been detected more frequently in Crohn's patients tissues, blood, and even breast milk compared to healthy controls. Studies show odds ratios as high as 7:1 for MAP presence in Crohn's versus controls, suggesting a strong association. Animal models and cell wall deficient forms of MAP isolated from human tissues further bolster this link, implying that MAP could trigger the granulomatous inflammation hallmark of Crohn's.

However, acceptance has been stymied. Critics point to inconsistent detection methods, such as PCR tests prone to false positives or negatives and cultures taking months, as reasons to dismiss it. More damningly, MAP fails Kochs postulates, the gold standard for proving bacterial causation, due to ethical impossibilities: you cannot infect children with MAP and wait 15 years to observe Crohn's development. As microbiologist Michael T. Collins notes, direct evidence that MAP causes Crohn's is impossible to obtain, as it would be unethical to infect very young children with MAP, wait 15 years, and see what happens. This ethical hurdle is weaponized to downplay the hypothesis, ignoring indirect evidence like higher MAP prevalence and successful antibiotic trials.

Governmental agencies compound this suppression. No body, whether the USDA or CDC, has declared MAP a zoonotic pathogen, citing only indirect evidence. This reluctance halts public health measures, like testing food supplies, and starves research funding. In a system where biologics rake in $13 billion annually, pursuing a bacterial cure threatens the narrative of Crohn's as an incurable autoimmune disorder.

Manipulated Trials: The Case of the Selby Study

Perhaps the most egregious example of data manipulation comes from clinical trials on anti-MAP therapy (AMT). AMT uses antibiotic combinations like clarithromycin, rifabutin, and clofazimine to target MAP, showing promise in case series and randomized controlled trials (RCTs). Yet, key studies have been interpreted, or misinterpreted, to bury these findings.

The 2007 Selby et al. RCT, a double blind, placebo controlled trial of 213 Crohn's patients, initially concluded no sustained benefit from AMT beyond placebo. This study is frequently cited to refute the MAP hypothesis. However, a 2008 reanalysis by Behr et al. revealed flaws: the original per protocol analysis overlooked intention to treat data, which showed significant benefits at 12 and 24 months. Critics also noted suboptimal dosing, such as double encapsulated clofazimine potentially reducing bioavailability, and the lack of a true placebo arm, skewing results.

This is not an isolated case. Earlier trials like Swift et al. (1994, 1998) used anti TB drugs ineffective against MAP, yielding no benefits and further discrediting AMT. Meanwhile, positive data from Borody et al. (2007) showed endoscopic healing in 56% of severe cases, and Gui et al. (1997) reported reduced corticosteroid use and improved indices after two years. The MAP US Phase III trial with RHB 104 demonstrated 37% remission at week 26 versus 23% placebo (p=0.007), with endoscopic improvements.

Why the discrepancies? Reanalyses suggest selective reporting: original conclusions downplay benefits, while follow ups uncover them. This pattern implies data removal through biased analysis, perpetuating skepticism. Guidelines from UK, US, and European bodies ignore AMT, citing lack of conclusive data, despite meta analyses favoring antibiotics like clofazimine.

Pharmaceutical Profits: Biologics Over Antibiotics
At the core of this suppression is economics. Biologics like Humira and Remicade generate billions, with Humira alone peaking at $20 billion, requiring lifelong use at $20,000 $85,000 annually. AMT, using off patent antibiotics, costs a fraction, potentially $1,000 $2,000 per course, and aims for cure, not management.

Pharmaceutical companies have little incentive to fund MAP research. RedHill Biopharmas RHB 104 and RHB 204 face hurdles despite positive data, with self-funding for off label AMT limiting access. The industry's focus on immunosuppression, effective but non curative, aligns with profit: why cure when you can treat indefinitely?

Interdisciplinary barriers exacerbate this. Gastroenterologists dominate, sidelining microbiologists and veterinarians needed for MAP expertise. Funding shortages and regulatory caution slow trials, as seen in the lack of large scale MAP studies despite 140 years of evidence.

Microbiota manipulation, like fecal microbiota transplantation (FMT), faces similar controversies. Challenges include donor variability, regulatory classification (drug versus tissue), and inconsistent outcomes, leading to underutilization. These hurdles mask potential cures, keeping patients dependent on high-cost drugs.

The Broader Implications: A Public Health Failure
The suppression of MAP related treatments extends beyond clinical trials to public health. MAPs presence in dairy products, water, and even breast milk raises alarms about zoonotic transmission. Studies estimate MAP in up to 20% of pasteurized milk samples, yet no regulatory body mandates testing or labeling. This inaction protects agribusiness interests, which contribute billions to economies, while ignoring risks to Crohn's patients and the broader population.

The failure to investigate MAP transmission mirrors the broader conspiracy. If Crohn's could be prevented through food safety measures or treated with antibiotics, the $13 billion Crohn's market would collapse. Instead, patients are funneled into a cycle of biologics, hospitalizations, and surgeries, with average annual costs of $10,000 $30,000 per patient. The global inflammatory bowel disease market, projected to hit $35.88 billion by 2034, thrives on this status quo.

Personal Reflections: The Cost of Concealed Knowledge
My journey with Crohn's has been a rollercoaster of hope and frustration. The epiphany in my adult years came when I stumbled upon MAP research, buried in

obscure journals and absent from doctor discussions. Switching to a plant based diet to avoid potential MAP sources brought some relief, but the question gnawed: why was this not mainstream knowledge? The suppressed data from trials like Selby fueled my anger. Had reanalyses been prioritized, perhaps my decades of flares, surgeries, and financial strain could have been mitigated.

This conspiracy is not abstract; it is in the denied funding, the twisted interpretations, the lives prolonged in pain. As an advocate now, I push for transparency: fund MAP trials, reform clinical guidelines, expose the profit driven veil. Every flare I endure, every bill I pay, is a reminder of the cures kept out of reach.

Community Voices: The Shared Struggle
The Crohn's community echoes my frustration. Online forums buzz with stories of patients discovering MAP research independently, only to face dismissive doctors. One patient wrote, I found Borodys work on anti-MAP therapy, but my GI laughed it off, saying it's not in the guidelines. Another shared spending $50,000 on biologics while reading about $1,000 antibiotic courses that could have helped. These voices, often silenced in clinical settings, fuel our collective resolve to unearth hidden treatments.

The Path Forward: Breaking the Silence
Breaking this conspiracy requires action. First, we need funding for independent MAP trials, free from pharmaceutical bias. Second, regulatory bodies must classify MAP as a zoonotic risk, mandating food and water testing. Third, clinical guidelines should

incorporate AMT and FMT, reflecting reanalyzed data. Finally, patients must advocate, sharing stories and demanding accountability.

The proof is there: reanalyzed trials, MAP detection studies, and patient outcomes. The Selby study's hidden benefits, the MAP US trials success, and decades of ignored correlations are not coincidences; they are evidence of suppression. As patients, we cannot wait for the system to self correct. We must push for the truth to be acknowledged.

The suppression of Crohn's treatments is not paranoia; it is evidenced in manipulated data, ethical excuses, and economic motives. From the Selby reanalysis to ignored MAP detections, the proof is clear: potential cures are hidden to preserve profits. As I stand with the Crohn's community, unbowed and unbroken, I call for unity to unearth these truths. We deserve treatments that heal, not just manage; we demand a system that prioritizes cures over cash. The conspiracy is real, but so is our resolve to end it, turning hidden hope into tangible healing.

Rod Chiodini:
A Pioneer's Legacy in Crohn's Research add in Lab destruction

In the labyrinth of Crohn's disease research, few names resonate as powerfully as Rod Chiodini's. A microbiologist whose work in the 1980s sparked a paradigm shift, Chiodini dared to challenge the conventional understanding of Crohn's as a purely autoimmune disorder. His hypothesis that *Mycobacterium avium subspecies paratuberculosis* (MAP), a bacterium linked to Johne's disease in cattle, could be a causative agent in Crohn's ignited both hope and controversy. For patients like me, grappling with the relentless symptoms of this chronic illness, Chiodini's work offered a tantalizing possibility: what if Crohn's wasn't just a genetic or immune misfire, but a treatable bacterial infection? This chapter delves into Chiodini's pioneering research, his tireless advocacy, the resistance he faced, and the profound implications of his findings for those of us living with Crohn's. His legacy is not just scientific it's a beacon for those seeking answers in a medical system often reluctant to embrace disruptive truths.

The Genesis of a Hypothesis
Rod Chiodini's journey into Crohn's research began in the early 1980s at the University of Connecticut Health Center, where he was a young microbiologist studying mycobacterial diseases. At the time, Crohn's disease was widely regarded as an autoimmune condition, its causes shrouded in mystery. Treatments focused on suppressing the immune system with drugs like corticosteroids or biologics, offering relief but no cure. Chiodini, however, saw parallels between Crohn's and Johne's disease, a chronic wasting condition in cattle caused by MAP. Both diseases shared eerie similarities: chronic inflammation of the intestines,

granulomatous lesions, and a relapsing remitting course. Could the same pathogen be at play?

In 1984, Chiodini and his team made a groundbreaking discovery. They successfully isolated MAP from the intestinal tissue of a Crohn's patient a 14 year old boy whose severe symptoms mirrored those of Johne's disease in livestock. This was no small feat. Mycobacteria are notoriously difficult to culture, requiring specialized techniques and patience. Chiodini's success, published in *Digestive Diseases and Sciences*, sent ripples through the medical community. For the first time, a tangible link between a specific pathogen and Crohn's disease had been established. The implications were staggering: if MAP was a cause, Crohn's might be treatable with antibiotics rather than lifelong immunosuppression.

Yet, the discovery was met with skepticism. The medical establishment, wedded to the autoimmune model, questioned the specificity of Chiodini's findings. Critics argued that MAP could be a secondary invader, present but not causative. Others pointed to the lack of consistent MAP detection across all Crohn's patients. Chiodini, undeterred, pressed forward, refining his methods and collaborating with researchers worldwide to build a stronger case.

Building the Case: Chiodini's Research Expands
By the late 1980s, Chiodini had moved to Rhode Island Hospital and Brown University, where he deepened his investigation into MAP's role in Crohn's. His work focused on three key areas: improving detection methods, understanding MAP's prevalence in Crohn's patients, and exploring therapeutic implications. At the

time, diagnostic tools for MAP were rudimentary. Standard cultures could take months, and early PCR techniques were not yet widely available. Chiodini developed innovative culturing methods, allowing for faster and more reliable detection of MAP in human tissue.

His studies revealed that MAP was present in a significant subset of Crohn's patients up to 50% in some cohorts compared to much lower rates in healthy controls or those with ulcerative colitis. This wasn't universal, which fueled debate, but Chiodini argued that Crohn's might not be a single disease but a spectrum of conditions with multiple triggers, MAP being one. His 1989 paper in *Journal of Clinical Microbiology* detailed these findings, emphasizing that MAP's slow growing nature and ability to persist in the body could explain the chronicity of Crohn's symptoms.

Chiodini's work also extended to animal models. He demonstrated that MAP could induce Crohn's like inflammation in goats and other species, providing a biological parallel to human disease. These experiments strengthened the hypothesis that MAP wasn't merely a bystander but a potential driver of intestinal inflammation. For patients like me, reading about these studies years later was a revelation. The idea that a bacterium could be at the root of my suffering offered a concrete target something to fight beyond the vague label of "autoimmune."

Collaboration and Controversy
Chiodini's research didn't occur in isolation. He collaborated with scientists like Saleh Naser at the

University of Central Florida, who advanced molecular techniques to detect MAP DNA in Crohn's patients' blood and tissue. Their joint work, published in journals like *The Lancet*, showed that MAP wasn't just present in the gut but could circulate systemically, potentially explaining extraintestinal symptoms like joint pain or fatigue. These findings aligned with my own experiences Crohn's wasn't confined to my gut; it affected my entire body, my energy, my life.

Yet, the MAP hypothesis faced fierce opposition. Pharmaceutical companies, heavily invested in biologics like anti TNF drugs, had little incentive to explore a bacterial cause that might shift treatment toward antibiotics. Regulatory bodies and funding agencies, too, were slow to support large scale MAP studies. Chiodini's critics argued that correlation didn't equal causation, and the absence of MAP in some patients suggested it wasn't the sole driver. The debate became a microcosm of the broader "conspiracy" I've come to see in Crohn's care: a system resistant to paradigm shifts, prioritizing profit and dogma over patient outcomes.

Chiodini's response was to double down on evidence. In the 1990s, he worked with international researchers, including those in Australia and Europe, to study MAP's prevalence in milk and water supplies. MAP's ability to survive pasteurization raised alarming questions about its transmission to humans, particularly through dairy products. This wasn't just a medical issue it was a public health concern. For me, learning that the food I consumed might harbor the very pathogen driving my disease was both infuriating and empowering. It fueled my resolve to question everything about Crohn's treatment.

The Therapeutic Frontier: MAP and Treatment
Perhaps Chiodini's most impactful contribution was his push for antibiotic therapies targeting MAP. If Crohn's was, in part, an infectious disease, then antimicrobials could offer a path to remission or even cure. Chiodini's team explored combinations of drugs like rifabutin, clarithromycin, and clofazimine antibiotics known to combat mycobacterial infections like tuberculosis. Early clinical trials, though small, showed promise. Some patients experienced significant symptom relief, and a few achieved long term remission.

These findings resonated deeply with me. In my own journey, I'd grown weary of steroids and biologics that dulled my symptoms but left me vulnerable to infections and side effects. The idea of targeting a root cause, rather than masking symptoms, felt like a lifeline. Chiodini's work inspired researchers like Thomas Borody, whose antibiotic protocols built on these ideas. Borody's success with anti-MAP therapy in Australia validated Chiodini's hypothesis, though mainstream adoption remained elusive.

The resistance to antibiotic trials wasn't just scientific it was systemic. Large scale studies required funding, and pharmaceutical giants weren't keen to invest in cheap, off patent drugs. Regulatory hurdles, too, slowed progress. Chiodini's advocacy for patients became as critical as his lab work. He spoke at conferences, engaged with patient groups, and pushed for more research, urging the medical community to take MAP seriously. His persistence reminded me of my own fight unbowed, unbroken.

St. Vincent Healthcare and Beyond

In later years, Chiodini's work found a new home at St. Vincent Healthcare in Montana, where he served as a consulting microbiologist. There, he focused on improving diagnostic tools for MAP, collaborating with clinicians to integrate his findings into patient care. His efforts at St. Vincent emphasized practical outcomes: better tests, faster diagnoses, and tailored treatments. For patients, this meant hope, hope that their disease could be understood and managed with precision.

Chiodini's work at St. Vincent also highlighted a broader issue: the gap between research and clinical practice. Even as evidence for MAP's role mounted, many gastroenterologists remained unaware or dismissive. This disconnect, which I've felt in countless doctor's appointments, underscored the "conspiracy" at the heart of this book. Why were promising leads like Chiodini's sidelined? Why did patients have to fight for access to therapies backed by decades of research?

Personal Reflections: Chiodini's Impact on My Journey

As I reflect on Chiodini's work, I'm struck by its personal significance. In my teens and young adult years, I accepted the standard narrative of Crohn's as an autoimmune disease. But reading about MAP in my adult years around the time of my epiphany changed everything. Chiodini's hypothesis gave me a framework to question the treatments I'd been prescribed, the food I ate, and the system that shaped my care. His courage in facing skepticism mirrored my own resolve to challenge the status quo.

I've never met Chiodini, but his work feels like a conversation across time. When I learned that MAP might be in milk, I switched to plant based alternatives, a small act of agency inspired by his findings. When I read about antibiotic trials, I sought out doctors willing to explore them, even if it meant traveling far from home. Chiodini's legacy isn't just in journals it's in the choice's patients like me make, the questions we ask, and the hope we hold.

The Broader Implications: A Call to Action

Chiodini's work raises profound questions about Crohn's and the medical system. If MAP is a cause, why hasn't it been prioritized? The answer lies in the interplay of profit, inertia, and fear of change. Pharmaceutical companies profit billions from biologics, while antibiotics like rifabutin are inexpensive and off patent. Regulatory agencies, cautious by nature, demand exhaustive evidence, even as patients suffer. And the public health implications MAP in food and water require political will that's hard to muster.

Yet, Chiodini's legacy is one of possibility. His research suggests that Crohn's might be preventable or treatable for some, if not all, patients. It challenges us to demand more from science and medicine to fund MAP studies, to test our food supply, to listen to patients. Chiodini's work isn't just a scientific footnote; it's a rallying cry.

Rod Chiodini's contributions to Crohn's research are a cornerstone of the fight for answers. His discovery of MAP's link to Crohn's, his persistence in the face of skepticism, and his advocacy for patients have reshaped the conversation around this disease. For those of us living with Crohn's, his work offers hope and a challenge: to question, to push, to demand better. As I continue my journey, documented in these pages, I carry Chiodini's legacy with me a reminder that truth, though hard won, is worth pursuing. In a world where medical conspiracies too often silence pioneers, Chiodini stands as a beacon, unbowed and unbroken.

THOMAS BORODY:
Patents, Trademarks, and the Fight for Crohn's Innovation

In the relentless battle against Crohn's disease, few names shine as brightly or spark as much controversy as Professor Thomas J. Borody. A gastroenterologist, innovator, and director of the Centre for Digestive Diseases (CDD) in Sydney, Australia, Borody has spent decades challenging the status quo of gastrointestinal treatment. His work, introduced in the Borody chapter, revolutionized our understanding of Crohn's through therapies like fecal microbiota transplantation (FMT) and anti Mycobacterium avium subspecies paratuberculosis (MAP) protocols. But behind these medical breakthroughs lies a vast portfolio of over 180 patents and trademarks, a testament to his drive to transform patient care. These intellectual properties, spanning FMT, antibiotic combinations, and novel delivery systems, are not just scientific milestones they're battlegrounds in a war against a medical establishment often resistant to disruptive cures. This chapter explores Borody's patents and trademarks, their implications for Crohn's patients like me, the controversies they've ignited, and their role in the broader "Crohn's Conspiracy" where profit and inertia stifle innovation. As I've learned through my own journey, Borody's work offers hope, but it also exposes the systemic barriers we face.

Borody's work is potentially as revolutionary as the discovery in 1984 that Peptic Ulcers were caused by a bacteria rather than stress or acid, so they could be cured with antibiotics.

Centre For Digestive Diseases (prof Borody) treats patients with Crohn's Disease using a novel approach of antibiotics designed to attack the underlying infection which we believe causes the disease. Instead of treating inflammation, we're treating an infection which is causing the inflammation.

Center For Digestive Diseases Professor Tom Borody

Professor Borody is most famous for his ground-breaking work developing the triple therapy cure for peptic ulcers in 1987 which has saved hundreds of thousands of lives, and the Australian health system more than $10 billion in medical care and operations and Professor Borody founded the Centre for Digestive Diseases (CDD) in 1984 after a distinguished career with leading hospitals including St Vincent's in Sydney and the Mayo Clinic in the USA.

He is a world-renowned leader in the clinical microbiota field dating back to 1988 when he started performing what is now called Fecal Microbiota Transplantation (FMT).

Professor Borody holds over 180 patents in areas such as; treatment of Helicobacter pylori, Crohn's disease, bowel lavage, IBS and FMT.

Fecal Microbiota Transplantation (FMT)

As a practicing clinician leading the CDD in Australia, Professor Borody has overseen over 14,000 FMTs, creating a wealth of proprietary clinical data and insights.

Inflammatory disease and infection.

In addition, Professor Borody has established novel therapies in the gastrointestinal field, including areas such as inflammatory bowel disease (IBD), irritable bowel syndrome (IBS), Clostridium difficile Infection (CDI), parasite infestation, and resistant Helicobacter pylori [1].

Peer review

His knowledge and expertise are sought after by clinicians from around the world. He is a reviewer for leading medical journals including:

• Journal of Clinical Gastroenterology • World Journal of Gastrointestinal Pharmacology and Therapeutics

• American Journal of Gastroenterology • Journal of Digestive Diseases and Sciences • Journal of Endoscopy

• Journal of Gastroenterology and Hepatology • Medical Journal of Australia

• Journal of Digestive and Liver Diseases • Helicobacter

Prof. Borody has over 200 articles and abstracts. His knowledge and expertise have been sought after by patients from around the world. The results have seen Prof. Borody become a reviewer for esteemed medical journals such as the Medical Journal of Australia, the American Journal of Gastroenterology, Journal of Gastroenterology and Hepatology, Digestive and Liver Diseases, J Clinical Gastroenterology and others.

Prof. Borody has established novel therapies in gastrointestinal areas such as Inflammatory Bowel Disease, Irritable Bowel Syndrome, Parasite infestation, Pesistant Helicobacter pylori and C. difficile.

The Foundation: Borody's Early Innovations

Thomas Borody's journey as an inventor began in the 1980s, a period when Crohn's was firmly entrenched as an autoimmune mystery, treated with crude tools like steroids and surgery. Born in Krakow in 1950 and trained at the University of New South Wales, Borody's exposure to parasitology and mycobacterial diseases in the Solomon Islands sparked a lifelong curiosity about gut infections. His time at the Mayo Clinic and subsequent degrees (MD, PhD, DSc) honed a rigorous approach to clinical research, leading to his establishment of the CDD in 1984.

Borody's first major breakthrough came in 1985 with a triple antibiotic therapy for *Helicobacter pylori*, the bacterium linked to peptic ulcers. This combination bismuth, tetracycline, and metronidazole cured patients where surgery once loomed, earning global acclaim and commercialization as Helidac in the U.S. Later, he licensed a quadruple therapy, Pylera, and a next generation treatment for resistant *H. pylori*, Talicia, to RedHill Biopharma. These successes, patented early in his career, set the stage for his approach: identify a microbial culprit, develop targeted therapies, and protect them via intellectual property to ensure clinical adoption.

By 2025, Borody holds over 180 patents, many focused on gastrointestinal disorders like Crohn's, ulcerative colitis, and irritable bowel syndrome (IBS). His patents, cataloged on platforms like Justia and Google Patents, cover compositions, methods, and devices, reflecting a multifaceted strategy to address chronic diseases. Trademarks, such as Ziverdox for a controversial COVID 19 therapy, further illustrate his knack for branding innovations. For Crohn's patients, his work on FMT and anti-MAP therapies stands out, promising alternatives to the lifelong dependency fostered by biologics.

Pioneering FMT: Patents That Redefine Gut Health
Borody's most transformative contribution to Crohn's research is his pioneering use of FMT, a therapy he began exploring in 1988. FMT involves transplanting healthy donor fecal microbes into a patient's gut to restore a balanced microbiome, addressing conditions like *Clostridioides difficile* infection (CDI) and, potentially, Crohn's. His first FMT patient, treated for colitis, remains symptom free over 25 years later a powerful anecdote that fueled his patent pursuits.

Key FMT patents include US8460648B2 and WO2002007741A1, both titled "Probiotic Recolonisation Therapy." Filed in 2001 and granted in 2013 and later, these patents describe compositions of non pathogenic or attenuated microbes (e.g., *Clostridia*, *Bacteroides*, *E. coli*) for treating chronic gut disorders, including Crohn's, ulcerative colitis, and IBS. The compositions aim to correct abnormal microflora distributions, offering a radical departure from immunosuppressive drugs. Another patent, US5443826A (granted 1995, expired 2012), outlines methods for replacing diseased gut flora with healthy fecal flora, a precursor to modern FMT protocols.

Borody's FMT patents are expansive, covering formulations for gastric, gastrointestinal, and colonic treatments, including storage methods for long term stability at ambient temperatures (US10463702, US11207356). These innovations address practical barriers, enabling scalable, accessible therapies. At the CDD, Borody has overseen nearly 14,000 FMT procedures, generating proprietary data that strengthens his intellectual property claims. For me, discovering FMT in my adult years around the epiphany described in the first part of this book was a revelation. The idea that my gut's ecosystem could be rebuilt, not just suppressed, offered a lifeline beyond the biologics treadmill.

Yet, these patents face challenges. FMT's reliance on donor material raises regulatory hurdles, as agencies like the FDA classify it variably as a drug, biologic, or tissue. Borody's compositions, patented to include specific microbial strains, aim to standardize FMT, but commercialization lags. Why? The answer lies in economics: FMT, especially using affordable donor material, threatens the $13 billion Crohn's market dominated by biologics like Humira. Patents, while protective, require funding to translate into products a hurdle Borody navigates through partnerships like Crestovo Holdings.

Anti MAP Therapies: Patents Challenging the Autoimmune Paradigm
Borody's work on MAP, building on Rod Chiodini's discoveries, is another cornerstone of his patent

portfolio. Recognizing parallels between Crohn's and Johne's disease in cattle, Borody developed antibiotic combinations targeting MAP as a potential Crohn's trigger. His collaboration with RedHill Biopharma led to therapies like RHB 104, now advancing as RHB 204. These efforts are backed by patents like WO2017143386A1 (filed 2017), which covers compositions using *Dietzia* bacteria and other Actinobacteria to treat chronic infections, including MAP related Crohn's.

These patents propose methods to eradicate MAP, which Borody and co inventors argue persists in Crohn's patients, driving inflammation. A pivotal trial, now in late stages, tests a triple antibiotic regimen (rifabutin, clarithromycin, clofazimine) for Crohn's, showing remission rates surpassing standard care. Borody's intellectual property also includes formulations for bowel lavage and orthostatic cleansing (US10463702, US11207356), used to prepare patients for FMT or antibiotic therapy, enhancing efficacy.

The significance for Crohn's patients is profound. As I learned about MAP in my research, the possibility of targeting a root cause rather than masking symptoms reshaped my approach to treatment. Borody's patents, by protecting these methods, aim to bring them to market, but resistance is fierce. Pharmaceutical giants, profiting from biologics costing $20,000 $85,000 annually, have little incentive to fund studies of off patent antibiotics costing a fraction of that. Regulatory bodies, cautious about long term antibiotic use, demand exhaustive trials, delaying adoption. This tension between innovation and inertia mirrors the "conspiracy" I've felt in my own care, where promising therapies are sidelined.

Trademarks: Branding the Future of Treatment

Borody's trademarks complement his patents, creating recognizable brands for his therapies. The most notable is Ziverdox, a trademarked COVID 19 treatment combining ivermectin, doxycycline, and zinc, patented in December 2020 and licensed to Topelia Australia. Announced in 2021, Ziverdox sparked controversy when Borody promoted it without disclosing his patent interest, raising ethical questions about conflicts of interest. The Guardian reported that Borody's failure to declare potential profits while lobbying Australian officials exemplified the murky intersection of science and commerce.

While Ziverdox isn't directly Crohn's related, it reflects Borody's broader approach: develop innovative therapies, protect them legally, and push for adoption, even against skepticism. His other trademarks, less publicized, likely cover formulations or devices at the CDD, such as Glycoprep and Moviprep, colonoscopy bowel prep products licensed to Salix. These trademarks ensure market exclusivity, critical for funding further research but also a flashpoint for critics who see profiteering.

For me, the Ziverdox controversy was a wake-up call. It highlighted how even pioneers like Borody navigate a system where intellectual property can both drive and derail progress. The Crohn's community, desperate for solutions, doesn't care about patents we want results. Yet, Borody's trademarks underscore a harsh reality: without legal protections, innovations risk being buried by larger players.

The Autism Connection: Expanding the Patent Horizon

Borody's patents extend beyond Crohn's, notably into autism spectrum disorder (ASD), where gut microbiota imbalances are implicated. Patents like those co invented with James Adams and others (filed with Arizona State University and Finch Therapeutics) describe FMT based treatments for ASD, with or without gastrointestinal symptoms. These patents outline protocols involving antibiotics, bowel cleansing, and purified fecal microbiota, aiming to restore healthy gut flora and alleviate neurological symptoms.

This work resonates with Crohn's research, as both conditions involve microbiome dysregulation. Borody's ASD patents suggest a unified theory: chronic diseases, from Crohn's to autism, may stem from microbial imbalances treatable through targeted interventions. For patients, this offers a holistic perspective my Crohn's flares often coincide with cognitive fog, hinting at gut brain connections Borody's patents explore.

However, these patents face similar barriers: regulatory complexity and industry preference for symptom focused drugs. The ASD market, like Crohn's, is lucrative, with behavioral therapies and medications generating billions. FMT, though promising, struggles for mainstream acceptance, leaving Borody's innovations in a holding pattern.

Systemic Barriers: The Conspiracy at Play

Borody's patents and trademarks reveal a deeper truth about the Crohn's landscape: innovation is only as impactful as the system allows. The pharmaceutical industry, with its $35.88 billion IBD market forecast by 2034, thrives on chronicity. Biologics like Remicade and Humira, costing patients $20,000 $85,000 yearly, ensure steady revenue. Borody's solutions FMT costing thousands per course, or antibiotics under $2,000 threaten this model. His patents, while robust, require partners like RedHill or Finch Therapeutics to navigate clinical trials and regulatory mazes, processes that drain resources.

The Ziverdox saga exemplifies this. Borody's advocacy for an unproven COVID 19 therapy, patented for profit, drew scrutiny for undeclared conflicts. Yet, this mirrors the Crohn's arena: promising therapies languish without funding, while approved drugs dominate through marketing muscle. Borody's 180+ patents, from FMT to bowel preps, face a system favoring high margin, patent protected biologics over affordable cures.

Public health implications add another layer. Borody's MAP related patents raise questions about dairy safety, as MAP survives pasteurization. Yet, agribusiness and regulatory inertia block widespread testing, protecting economic interests over patient health. This is the "conspiracy" I've felt in my own journey: a system that prioritizes profit over prevention, management over eradication.

Personal Reflections: Borody's Impact on My Fight

Borody's work has been a beacon in my Crohn's odyssey. From the despair of my young adult years to the epiphany of questioning autoimmune dogma, his FMT and anti-MAP therapies offered a new lens. I explored FMT after reading about his 1988 success, seeking clinics willing to try it. The financial burden thousands out of pocket paled compared to biologics, but access was limited. Borody's patents, meant to democratize these therapies, are caught in a web of resistance, mirroring my struggle to find doctors open to alternatives.

His story fuels my advocacy. If a pioneer with 180 patents faces pushback, what chance do patients have without collective action? I've joined forums, written to policymakers, and shared Borody's findings, urging funding for his trials. His trademarks, like Ziverdox, remind me that even well intentioned innovators must navigate a flawed system a system I'm determined to challenge.

Thomas Borody's patents and trademarks are more than legal documents; they're a blueprint for revolutionizing Crohn's care. From FMT's microbial restoration to anti MAP therapies targeting root causes, his intellectual property challenges a profit driven medical establishment. Yet, the slow march to adoption hampered by funding shortages, regulatory caution, and industry bias reveals the Crohn's Conspiracy at its core. For patients like me, Borody's work is a lifeline, a call to question, innovate, and fight. As we stand unbowed and unbroken, his legacy inspires us to demand a future where cures, not profits, define our care.

THE WORK OF JOHN AITKEN
OTAKARO PATHWAYS NEW ZEALAND

John Aitken, a dedicated microbiologist based in Christchurch, New Zealand, has devoted over four decades to unraveling the mysteries of bacterial infections, with a particular focus on Crohn's disease and its potential link to Mycobacterium avium subspecies paratuberculosis (MAP). As the senior director of Otakaro Pathways, Ltd., Aitken has emerged as a leading figure in MAP research, driven by a personal brush with Crohn's like symptoms at age 23 and a deep empathy for those affected by the chronic illness, especially the "Crohn's mothers" who advocate for their children's health. His work blends rigorous science with a commitment to finding practical solutions for patients suffering from this debilitating condition.

Aitken's journey into Crohn's research began with a personal health scare that sharpened his curiosity about the disease's origins. Over the years, his expertise in medical microbiology honed through work with public and private providers led him to investigate MAP, a bacterium known to cause Johne's disease in livestock, which shares striking similarities with Crohn's in humans. At Otakaro Pathways, Aitken and his team achieved a scientific breakthrough by developing a diagnostic test to detect MAP in human blood, a challenging task due to the bacterium's elusive, cell wall deficient form. This test, priced at $250 USD, has provided hundreds of patients including myself with insights into their condition, empowering them to explore targeted treatments like anti- MAP antibiotic therapy.

Beyond the lab, Aitken's advocacy is fueled by stories of families grappling with Crohn's, particularly parents desperate for answers. He has collaborated with global researchers, including Australia's Dr. Thomas Borody, to study anti-MAP antibiotics, which show remission rates of 8090% in some cases. Aitken's holistic approach emphasizing the bacterium's life cycle and environmental interactions has challenged mainstream views that Crohn's is purely autoimmune, pushing for a bacterial trigger like MAP. Aitken's work is ongoing and is always collecting data and doing research, John Aitken continues to drive debate and hope for a cure for us all around the world.

PROJECT CENSORED
The Hidden Crisis of Foodborne Illness in the U.S.

In the sprawling web of America's food system, where glossy supermarket aisles hide gritty truths, a silent crisis festers: foodborne pathogens that may drive diseases like Crohn's are swept under the rug. For decades, I've battled Crohn's, a relentless illness that's been framed as an autoimmune enigma. But what if its roots lie in the milk we drink, the water we sip, or the meat we consume? This chapter, inspired by the investigative spirit of Project Censored, exposes how foodborne illnesses, particularly those linked to *Mycobacterium avium subspecies paratuberculosis* (MAP), are downplayed by a system prioritizing profit over health. MAP, a bacterium tied to Crohn's and found in dairy and water, survives pasteurization, yet regulatory bodies and agribusiness giants resist testing or action. The stakes are staggering: millions face chronic diseases, with Crohn's costing patients $10,000 $30,000 yearly, while the $13 billion inflammatory bowel disease market thrives on symptom management, not cures. Drawing on suppressed studies, whistleblower accounts, and my own journey, we'll uncover how data on MAP's risks is buried, leaving patients in the dark. This is not just a health issue; it's a conspiracy of silence, where economic interests mute the truth about what's on our plates, fueling a hidden epidemic that demands exposure.

REHASH OF THE PAPER THAT SAVED MY LIFE
A Readaptation from Michael Greger, MD; Originally written January 2001.

Project Censored: The Hidden Crisis of Foodborne Illness in the U.S.

Microbial foodborne illnesses remain the largest class of emerging infectious diseases worldwide, posing a significant and growing threat to public health. In 1999, the Centers for Disease Control and Prevention (CDC) released what the Food and Drug Administration (FDA) considered the most comprehensive estimate ever compiled on the incidence of foodborne illness in the United States.

The Alarming Statistics of Foodborne Illness

The CDC's findings revealed a disturbing reality:

- An estimated 76 million Americans contract food poisoning each year more than double previous estimates.
- In the U.S., the odds are startling:
  - 1 in 4 chance of getting sick from contaminated food annually.
  - 1 in 840 chance of being hospitalized.
  - 1 in 55,000 chance of dying from foodborne illness every year.

These numbers highlight the serious and often underappreciated threat that foodborne pathogens pose to the general population.

Animal Products: The Primary Source of Contamination

The CDC estimates that approximately 97% of foodborne illnesses are caused by animal based foods. According to a U.S. Department of Agriculture (USDA) survey:

- 90% of Thanksgiving turkeys were found to be contaminated with Campylobacter, the most common bacterial cause of food poisoning in the U.S.
- 75% of turkeys carried two or more foodborne pathogens, including Salmonella, which is becoming increasingly resistant to many of our most effective antibiotics.

This resistance makes foodborne infections harder to treat and increases the risk of severe complications.

Beyond Acute Illness: Long Term Complications

While most food poisoning cases resolve after a brief illness, the long term consequences can be severe:

- Up to 15% of individuals who contract Salmonella develop chronic joint inflammation, a condition known as reactive arthritis, which can last for years.
- An estimated 100,000 to 200,000 Americans each year suffer from arthritis directly caused by foodborne infections.

One of the most feared complications, however, is Guillain Barré syndrome:

- Triggered by Campylobacter infections, this rare autoimmune condition can cause paralysis and may require months of mechanical ventilation for survival.

- Approximately 3,800 cases are linked to Campylobacter infections annually in the U.S.

The Censored Crisis: Crohn's Disease and MAP in Milk

Beyond the known dangers of common foodborne pathogens, scientists are now raising alarms about a potentially even more serious and less acknowledged threat:

- Research suggests a possible connection between Crohn's disease and Mycobacterium avium subspecies paratuberculosis (MAP), a bacterium found in milk from cows infected with Johne's disease.
- This connection, despite growing scientific evidence, has received little mainstream attention.

In recognition of the media silence around this issue, the investigation into the link between Crohn's disease and MAP contamination received a Project Censored Award in 1999 often referred to as the Pulitzer Prize of alternative journalism.

A Growing Threat Ignored

The lack of public awareness surrounding foodborne illnesses particularly the potential connection between dairy consumption and chronic diseases like Crohn's reflects a troubling failure of both media coverage and government oversight. Despite growing scientific consensus, regulatory action remains minimal, and industry influence continues to suppress open dialogue on the issue.

Addressing this hidden crisis will require:

- Increased public awareness.
- Stricter food safety regulations.

- Transparent government action to protect consumers from emerging foodborne pathogens like MAP.

Until these measures are taken, millions of Americans remain at risk of both acute infections and chronic illnesses linked to contaminated food products.

Crohn's Disease: A Growing Health Crisis

Crohn's disease is a debilitating, lifelong condition that affects over half a million Americans and incurs annual healthcare costs totaling billions of dollars. Often described as a "human scourge", the disease relentlessly impacts the daily lives of its sufferers, with symptoms that can be both physically and emotionally devastating.

Living with Crohn's: A Daily Struggle

For those living with Crohn's, the symptoms can be relentless and life altering:
- Chronic episodes of urgent diarrhea, accompanied by nausea, vomiting, and fevers.
- Many sufferers become prisoners in their own homes due to the constant need for bathroom access. Others have resorted to using recreational vehicles or mobile homes to ensure they're always close to a restroom.
- As one expert from the National Association for Colitis and Crohn's Disease described it, living with Crohn's is like experiencing the worst stomach flu every single day.

A Disease That Attacks from Within

Crohn's disease is classified as an autoimmune disorder, meaning the body's immune system mistakenly attacks its own tissues:

- The immune response targets the lining of the digestive tract, causing inflammation and swelling.
- In severe cases, the disease can affect any part of the gastrointestinal system, from the mouth to the anus.
- The inflammation can narrow the digestive tract, leading to intense pain during digestion, uncontrollable bowel movements, and other complications such as:
  - Joint pain
  - Weight loss
  - Chronic fatigue

Physical Damage: The "Cobblestone" Gut

As Crohn's progresses, it can cause deep ulcerations in the intestinal walls, creating a characteristic "cobblestone" appearance:

- These ulcers can penetrate the intestinal wall, leading to:
  - Bleeding
  - Abscesses
  - Fistulas (abnormal connections between organs)
  - Perforations (holes in the gut wall)

One colorectal surgeon grimly referred to Crohn's as a "surgical disease", noting:

"We wait until the patient can no longer withstand the pain anymore, and then we perform surgery again and again until there's no intestine left to remove."

A Disease Striking the Young

One of the most heartbreaking aspects of Crohn's disease is that it often strikes during adolescence or early adulthood:

- Many patients are diagnosed in their teens or early twenties, forcing them to confront the reality of chronic illness for the rest of their lives.
- Children and young adults endure not only physical pain but also the emotional toll of being in and out of hospitals throughout their formative years.

An Epidemic on the Rise

While Crohn's disease was once considered rare, its incidence has been increasing dramatically:

- In the U.S., cases have doubled, then tripled, and are now approaching epidemic levels since the 1940s.
- The most alarming increase has been observed in children:
    - In the 1940s and 1950s, there were virtually no recorded cases of Crohn's in teenagers.
    - Today, 1 in 6 new cases are diagnosed in individuals under the age of 20.

A Growing Global Concern

Crohn's disease is most prevalent in countries with industrialized agriculture, including:

- The United States
- The United Kingdom
- Scandinavia

The rise in cases has led many researchers to question the role of environmental factors, including dietary changes and potential exposure to pathogens like Mycobacterium avium subspecies paratuberculosis (MAP).

A Monster Unleashed

Dr. Burrill Crohn, who first described the disease in 1932, would later reflect on its alarming growth:
"From this small beginning, we have witnessed the evolution of a Frankenstein monster."

With the rising number of cases and mounting evidence of environmental triggers, Crohn's disease has evolved from a rare medical curiosity into a pressing public health crisis one that demands urgent attention, research, and action.

Mycobacterium paratuberculosis: The Hidden Bacterial Threat

The bacterium responsible for Johne's disease a debilitating and chronic illness in cattle is known as Mycobacterium avium subspecies paratuberculosis (MAP). This elusive microbe has gained increasing attention from scientists due to its potential link to Crohn's disease in humans.

A Close Relative of Dangerous Pathogens

MAP belongs to the mycobacteria family, a group of bacteria infamous for causing serious diseases such as:

- Tuberculosis (TB)
- Leprosy

Before Heinrich Johne correctly identified MAP as a distinct pathogen in cattle, scientists believed that Johne's disease was simply a form of intestinal tuberculosis. The term "paratuberculosis" literally means "tuberculosis like", reflecting the similarities between the two diseases in both appearance and symptoms.

An Enigmatic and Elusive Pathogen
Despite decades of research, MAP remains one of the most puzzling bacteria known to science:

- It resides inside the host's cells but does not produce any known toxins or directly damage cells in the way many other pathogens do.
- The real harm comes from the host's immune response similar to diseases like hepatitis where the body attacks its own tissues in an effort to target the hidden bacteria.

In cattle, this immune reaction leads to Johne's disease, a chronic intestinal illness characterized by severe diarrhea, weight loss, and eventually death. The question that has baffled researchers for years is whether MAP could trigger a similar immune driven condition in humans.

MAP's Suspected Link to Crohn's Disease
Though MAP's role in cattle disease is well established, its potential connection to Crohn's disease remains a subject of intense debate:

- Some scientists argue that MAP could be a causative factor behind Crohn's disease, triggering an immune attack on the intestinal lining similar to how it affects cattle.
- Others believe that MAP might exploit the already damaged gut tissue in Crohn's patients, making it an opportunistic invader rather than the root cause.

The Urgent Need for Research

The possibility that MAP could be responsible for at least some cases of Crohn's disease has far reaching implications:

- If confirmed, it could lead to new treatment strategies, including targeted antibiotics that specifically eliminate MAP from the gut.
- It would also necessitate stricter controls in the dairy and meat industries to prevent the transmission of MAP from animals to humans.

Until definitive answers emerge, the link between Mycobacterium avium paratuberculosis and Crohn's disease remains one of the most urgent and controversial mysteries in modern medical research a hidden bacterial threat that could reshape our understanding of chronic gut illnesses.

Spheroplasts: The Hidden Form of MAP and Its Potential Link to Crohn's Disease

Mycobacterium avium subspecies paratuberculosis (MAP) is a highly adaptable bacterium, capable of causing chronic intestinal disease in a wide range of animals, including cattle, sheep, deer, rabbits, baboons, and even other primates. Given its ability to infect such a broad spectrum of species, scientists have long suspected that MAP might also pose a threat to humans.

The Elusive Nature of MAP in Humans

One of the key challenges in confirming MAP's role in Crohn's disease lies in the difficulty of detecting the bacterium in human tissue:

- In cattle suffering from Johne's disease, MAP is easy to visualize under a light microscope using

an acid fast stain a technique that highlights the bacteria's thick, waxy cell wall.
- However, when researchers attempted to find MAP in the intestinal tissues of Crohn's patients, they consistently failed to detect the familiar acid fast bacilli.

This discrepancy puzzled scientists for decades, as they struggled to understand why MAP was so easily identifiable in animals but seemingly invisible in humans.

The Discovery of Spheroplasts: A Breakthrough
The mystery remained unsolved until 1984, when microbiologist Rodrick Chiodini of Brown University's Rhode Island Hospital made a groundbreaking discovery:
- Chiodini successfully cultured live MAP bacteria from the intestinal walls of children suffering from Crohn's disease.
- His research revealed that MAP can exist in a "cell wall deficient" form, known as a spheroplast.

Why Spheroplasts Are So Hard to Detect
Spheroplasts represent a stealthy survival strategy for MAP:
- In this form, the bacterium sheds its cell wall, the very structure that would normally absorb the acid fast stain used to detect it.
- Without the cell wall, MAP becomes invisible under traditional staining methods used to identify mycobacterial infections.

Even more concerning, MAP has the ability to regrow its cell wall:

- Years after becoming a spheroplast, MAP can revert back to its typical form, making detection possible again.
- This transformation was confirmed in Chiodini's lab, where previously undetectable MAP bacteria later regenerated their cell walls and were successfully cultured.

The Spheroplast Hypothesis: Triggering Crohn's Disease?

Researchers now believe that these cell wall deficient forms of MAP may be responsible for triggering the abnormal immune response seen in Crohn's disease:

- Because MAP hides inside human cells without its cell wall, the immune system struggles to detect and eliminate the bacterium.
- Over time, the body's attempts to destroy the hidden pathogen can lead to chronic inflammation of the intestinal lining an autoimmune reaction that mirrors the symptoms of Crohn's disease.

A New Perspective on Crohn's Disease

The discovery of spheroplasts offers a compelling explanation for why:

- MAP is so difficult to detect in patients with Crohn's.
- Standard diagnostic tools fail to reveal its presence.
- Crohn's disease may be linked to a chronic, hidden infection that evades the immune system's usual defenses.

This research opens new possibilities for better diagnostic methods and targeted treatment strategies, focusing on eradicating the elusive spheroplast form of MAP potentially offering new hope for those suffering from this life altering disease.

Live Cultures: The Challenge of Growing MAP from Crohn's Patients

One of the most persistent challenges in unraveling the connection between Mycobacterium avium subspecies paratuberculosis (MAP) and Crohn's disease has been the difficulty of consistently culturing the bacterium from the intestinal tissue of those affected. Despite evidence suggesting a potential link, isolating and growing MAP from human samples has proven to be an extraordinarily difficult task.

A Global Effort with Inconsistent Results

Scientists across the world have attempted to isolate MAP from the tissues of Crohn's patients:

- Research centers in California, Texas, France, Australia, England, the Netherlands, and the Czech Republic have all reported successfully culturing MAP.
- However, results have been inconsistent and sparse many laboratories have failed to isolate the bacterium at all.

This inconsistency has led to skepticism within the scientific community about MAP's role in Crohn's disease. Yet, this failure isn't entirely surprising given the extreme difficulty involved in culturing MAP from human tissues.

Why Is Culturing MAP So Difficult?

There are several reasons why isolating MAP from human intestines presents such a challenge:

- Complex gut environment: The intestines are home to billions of bacteria, making it difficult to isolate MAP from this microbial jungle.
- Decontamination difficulties: Removing other bacteria without harming MAP requires precise and delicate techniques.
- Spheroplasts: When MAP sheds its cell wall (becoming a spheroplast), it becomes nearly impossible to grow in a lab using standard culturing techniques, as the methods used to kill off other bacteria also damage MAP in its weakened form.

The Time Consuming Process of Culturing MAP
Even if MAP survives the decontamination process, growing it in a lab is a slow and painstaking effort:
- Some cultures have taken up to six years to grow, even under highly controlled laboratory conditions.
- Rodrick Chiodini, who made a landmark breakthrough in culturing MAP from Crohn's patients, succeeded largely due to his years of experience and access to modern culture techniques.

Earlier researchers likely failed because they didn't meet the high standards now recognized as necessary for successful cultivation:
- Using fresh resected tissue (removed during surgery) has been found to be more effective than using older, frozen, or fixed samples.
- MAP tends to embed itself deep within the intestinal wall, meaning superficial biopsies often miss the bacteria altogether.

A Parallel to Other Elusive Pathogens
MAP isn't the only pathogen that has proven difficult to culture:

- The bacterium responsible for leprosy (*Mycobacterium leprae*) has never been successfully grown in a laboratory setting.
- Campylobacter, now known as a major cause of food poisoning, wasn't identified until the 1970s when culturing technology advanced enough to isolate it reliably.

Why So Few MAP Bacteria Might Still Cause Disease
Another complication is the sparse presence of MAP in Crohn's patients:

- In both humans and animals (like sheep and goats with paratuberculosis), the number of detectable MAP bacteria can be incredibly low.
- Similar to leprosy, even a small number of bacteria may be capable of triggering a severe immune response, leading to chronic inflammation and symptoms resembling Crohn's disease.

The Need for Better Culturing Techniques
Despite decades of effort, culturing MAP remains a significant hurdle in confirming its role in Crohn's disease:

- Current laboratory methods are often inconsistent or inadequate.
- Variations in research design across different labs have led to contradictory results.

Until new techniques are developed to reliably culture MAP from human tissue, this pathogen will remain difficult to study and its potential role in causing Crohn's disease will continue to be debated within the scientific community.

DNA Fingerprinting: A Breakthrough in Detecting MAP in Crohn's Disease
Culturing Mycobacterium avium subspecies paratuberculosis (MAP) from the tissues of Crohn's disease patients has long been a daunting task. The bacterium's elusive nature, especially in its cell wall deficient form (spheroplast), made it almost impossible to grow in laboratory conditions. However, the introduction of DNA fingerprinting technology in the late 1980s revolutionized researchers' ability to detect this hidden pathogen.

How DNA Fingerprinting Changed the Game
Instead of waiting months or even years for MAP to grow in a lab culture, scientists began using DNA probe technology, similar to methods used in forensic science, to detect even minute traces of MAP's genetic material:

- This technology allowed researchers to directly identify MAP's DNA in tissue samples, bypassing the need to grow live bacteria.
- It offered 100% certainty when MAP DNA was found, eliminating the need to wait for spheroplasts to revert to their normal, stainable form.

The Evidence: MAP DNA in Crohn's Patients

Using DNA fingerprinting, scientists made some striking discoveries:

- Approximately 65% of intestinal tissue samples from Crohn's disease patients tested positive for MAP DNA.
- By comparison, only 4% of samples from individuals with ulcerative colitis a disease with similar symptoms tested positive.

These findings provided compelling evidence of a potential connection between MAP and Crohn's disease, far stronger than previously possible using traditional culturing methods.

Challenges in Detecting MAP DNA

Despite these advancements, DNA fingerprinting isn't foolproof. Several factors complicate detection:

- Low bacterial concentration: MAP often exists in very small quantities, making it like searching for a needle in a haystack amid the billions of other bacterial DNA strands found in the gut.
- Interference by gut substances: Certain substances naturally present in the intestines, such as bile salts and polysaccharides, can inhibit the accuracy of DNA detection tests.
- Difficulty isolating MAP DNA: Mycobacterial DNA, in general, is notoriously challenging to extract due to the bacterium's tough and complex cell structure.

Diagnostic Uncertainty: Is It Always Crohn's?

Another challenge in establishing the MAP Crohn's connection is the issue of misdiagnosis:

- Studies suggest that up to 20% of patients diagnosed with Crohn's disease may actually be suffering from a different condition, such as ulcerative colitis.
- There is growing debate over whether Crohn's disease is even a single disease entity it may instead represent a collection of conditions with similar symptoms but differing causes, some unrelated to MAP altogether.

This uncertainty makes interpreting MAP DNA test results more complicated, as not all Crohn's patients will test positive for MAP.

MAP in Healthy Individuals: A Complex Puzzle

Interestingly, some individuals who do not have Crohn's disease also test positive for MAP:

- Exposure to MAP doesn't guarantee illness. For example, only about one third of calves exposed to MAP develop Johne's disease.
- It's possible that different strains of MAP exist, with some strains capable of causing disease and others remaining harmless.

The Key Takeaway: A Strong Association

Despite these complexities, the data reveal a consistently significant association:

- Studies across multiple continents have repeatedly found a strong link between the presence of Mycobacterium paratuberculosis and the development of Crohn's disease.
- While MAP may not be the sole cause of Crohn's, the evidence suggests it could play a central role in triggering or exacerbating the disease in genetically susceptible individuals.

As DNA fingerprinting techniques continue to evolve, they offer the potential for more accurate diagnostics, better treatment strategies, and a deeper understanding of how MAP may be contributing to one of the most challenging gastrointestinal diseases of our time.

Association or Causation? The MAP Crohn's Disease Debate

While Mycobacterium avium subspecies paratuberculosis (MAP) has been found far more frequently in the intestines of Crohn's disease patients than in those of healthy individuals, the central question remains:

Does MAP cause Crohn's disease, or is it simply an opportunistic invader of already inflamed tissue?

The Chicken or Egg Dilemma

Just because MAP is present in Crohn's sufferers doesn't necessarily mean it's the cause of the disease:

- Alternative explanation: MAP could simply exploit the already damaged gut environment, colonizing areas of inflammation caused by another underlying condition.
- If MAP only targeted inflamed tissue, it would also be found more frequently in diseases similar to Crohn's, like ulcerative colitis. However, studies show this is not the case.
- Other nonspecific mycobacteria are distributed uniformly across people with Crohn's, ulcerative colitis, colon cancer, and even healthy individuals, suggesting a unique relationship between MAP and Crohn's.

This pattern suggests that the presence of MAP in Crohn's disease isn't just coincidental but potentially pathogenic.

Proving Causation: Koch's Postulates
In medicine, scientists often rely on Koch's postulates a set of criteria developed by Robert Koch in 1876 to prove whether a specific pathogen causes a disease:
1. The organism must be present in every case of the disease.
2. It must be isolated and grown in pure culture.
3. Introducing the organism into a healthy host should cause the disease.
4. The organism must be re isolated from the newly infected host.

While these postulates have served as the gold standard for proving causation, they are not always reliable for diseases affecting humans:
- Some diseases, such as leprosy (caused by *Mycobacterium leprae*), have never fully met these criteria, yet are universally accepted as infectious diseases.
- Ethical concerns also arise when intentionally infecting animals or humans for experimental proof.

MAP Satisfies Koch's Postulates in Animal Models
Despite the challenges of proving causation directly in humans, experiments using animal models have produced compelling evidence:
- Chickens infected with MAP strains isolated from Crohn's patients developed intestinal disease resembling Crohn's.

- In 1986, researchers infected infant goats with human derived MAP strains. The goats developed Crohn's like symptoms, and the same strain of bacteria was re isolated from their tissues.

These experiments demonstrate that MAP can indeed cause disease that mimics Crohn's in other species.

Why the Medical Community Remains Skeptical

Despite this evidence, the scientific and medical communities remain cautious:

- Past attempts to link Crohn's disease to other infectious agents such as chlamydia or measles have been disproven.
- As a result, researchers are understandably skeptical about embracing a new infectious theory without overwhelming proof.

However, unlike previous suspects, MAP is:

- The only organism that has been consistently cultured from Crohn's disease tissues.
- The only one capable of causing an identical disease in animals.

Antibody Testing: A New Frontier for Detection

One method doctors use to detect infectious diseases involves searching for antibodies produced by the immune system in response to the pathogen:

- For diseases like HIV, detecting antibodies is often more effective than testing for the virus itself.
- Researchers have searched for anti-MAP antibodies in Crohn's patients, but finding an antibody that is specific to MAP has proven difficult.

Recent developments, however, show promise:

- Certain antibodies believed to be unique to MAP have been found in 90% of Crohn's patients, compared to less than 10% in individuals with ulcerative colitis.
- This discovery opens the door for future diagnostic tools, including the potential for a blood test to confirm MAP exposure in Crohn's disease patients.

A Path Toward Prevention: Vaccines and Treatments
If MAP's role in Crohn's disease is definitively confirmed, the implications are enormous:

- Scientists could develop targeted vaccines to prevent infection.
- New treatments could focus on eliminating MAP from infected individuals, offering hope for those suffering from this painful, lifelong condition.

While the association between MAP and Crohn's disease appears increasingly strong, proving causation remains the key challenge. Ongoing research continues to push the boundaries of our understanding and may soon offer new ways to diagnose, treat, and possibly prevent this devastating illness.

Epidemiology: Exploring the Global Connection Between MAP and Crohn's Disease

Population studies offer intriguing clues about the potential link between *Mycobacterium avium* subspecies *paratuberculosis* (MAP) and Crohn's disease. Regions with high rates of Johne's disease in cattle often overlap with areas showing elevated rates of Crohn's disease primarily in milk drinking nations such as the United States, Canada, Australia, Europe, New Zealand, and parts of southern Africa. Interestingly, India, where milk is commonly boiled before consumption, reports significantly fewer cases of Crohn's disease.

However, inconsistencies remain. For example, Sweden, which maintains reportedly low rates of paratuberculosis in cattle, still experiences cases of Crohn's disease. Experts like Dr. Michael Collins suggest that no country is truly free of MAP; it's more likely that insufficient testing masks the disease's true prevalence.

Another puzzle is the urban rural divide. Crohn's disease is more commonly found in urban populations than in rural ones, even though dairy farmers, who have higher exposure to livestock, don't show disproportionately high rates. A similar pattern was observed historically with bovine tuberculosis transmitted through unpasteurized milk, which also spread more through commercial milk distribution in cities than directly among rural farmers.

The sharp rise in Crohn's cases up to a 4000% increase since the 1930s in places like Wales may coincide with intensified dairy farming practices and the consolidation of milk production. As dairy conglomerates pool milk from numerous farms, the potential for MAP contamination could increase, spreading the bacterium more widely and potentially contributing to the modern Crohn's epidemic.

The Case of Nick Barnes: A Human Link Between MAP and Crohn's Disease

Nick Barnes, a seemingly healthy 7 year old boy, developed a swollen lump on the side of his neck an infection later confirmed to be caused by Mycobacterium avium subspecies paratuberculosis (MAP). This marked the first clear cut case of MAP infecting a human and causing visible disease, providing direct evidence that the bacterium could cross the species barrier from animals to humans.

The significance of this finding deepened when, five years later, Barnes was diagnosed with Crohn's disease. This timeline of infection followed by the onset of Crohn's presents a compelling case for MAP's potential role as a trigger for the disease.

Despite this strong association, the medical community remained hesitant to accept MAP as a cause of Crohn's. Such resistance reflects a broader pattern seen in medical history, where groundbreaking discoveries like the role of *Helicobacter pylori* in causing stomach ulcers faced skepticism before eventually gaining acceptance. Barnes' case remains a pivotal example fueling the ongoing debate over MAP's role in Crohn's disease.

The H. pylori Parallel: Lessons for Understanding MAP and Crohn's Disease

For decades, stomach ulcers were thought to be the result of stress and excess stomach acid, leading to the immune system attacking the stomach lining. Treatments focused on managing symptoms through medications and surgery, much like current approaches for Crohn's disease.

This perspective changed dramatically in the 1980s when two Australian researchers, Drs. Barry Marshall and Robin Warren, isolated a bacterium called *Helicobacter pylori* (H. pylori) from the stomach lining. Their radical hypothesis suggested that ulcers were not caused by stress but by a bacterial infection. Despite initial ridicule from the medical community many believed no bacteria could survive stomach acid persistent research eventually proved them right. Marshall even went as far as drinking a vial of the bacteria to prove its pathogenic potential. Ultimately, the definitive evidence came when patients' ulcers were cured by antibiotic treatments, revolutionizing how the medical field understood and treated the condition.

Many scientists now see a striking parallel between the *H. pylori* story and the ongoing debate surrounding *Mycobacterium avium* subspecies *paratuberculosis* (MAP) and Crohn's disease. Just as *H. pylori* was the hidden trigger for immune attacks on the stomach lining, researchers suspect that MAP might be the underlying cause of immune system attacks on the intestinal lining in Crohn's disease.

However, MAP presents even greater challenges it's difficult to detect, almost impossible to grow in standard lab cultures, evades immune system detection, and resists treatment. As Dr. John Hermon Taylor, a leading advocate for the MAP Crohn's connection, points out: if the hypothesis proves correct, the consequences could be far more significant than economic losses in livestock farming. It could fundamentally reshape our understanding and treatment of Crohn's disease, just as *H. pylori* transformed ulcer management.

Targeting MAP in Crohn's Disease: The Antibiotic Breakthrough
Inspired by the success of treating *Helicobacter pylori* infections in ulcers, researchers turned their focus to treating Crohn's disease with antibiotics targeting *Mycobacterium avium* subspecies *paratuberculosis* (MAP). The logic was straightforward: if MAP contributes to Crohn's disease, then eliminating it might lead to a cure or significant remission.

Early Challenges in Treatment Attempts
Initial attempts to treat Crohn's with antibiotics were met with disappointment. Researchers mistakenly assumed that drugs effective against *Mycobacterium tuberculosis* would also work against MAP an assumption that turned out to be incorrect. MAP proved resistant to traditional tuberculosis drugs, both in livestock and humans.

Further complicating these early efforts:
- Monotherapy Missteps: Early trials used single antibiotics, which are often ineffective against mycobacterial diseases since these bacteria easily develop resistance.
- Treatment Duration: Mycobacterial infections typically require long term, multi drug regimens. Treatments for related infections, such as leprosy, can span years yet early MAP trials were too short to be effective.

A Scientific Turning Point

The breakthrough came in 1992 when laboratory testing identified clarithromycin, a macrolide antibiotic, as highly effective against MAP. Unlike earlier treatments that targeted cell wall synthesis (ineffective against MAP's spheroplast form, which lacks a cell wall), clarithromycin worked by blocking protein synthesis. Another antibiotic, rifabutin, was found to be similarly effective.

Why did these drugs work when others failed?
- Intracellular Access: MAP hides inside human cells, making it difficult to target. Macrolides like clarithromycin can penetrate these cells and act directly on the bacteria.
- Multi Drug Strategies: Later treatment protocols combined multiple antibiotics to prevent bacterial resistance and ensure a more thorough eradication of the pathogen.

Complexities in Clinical Trials

Even with promising antibiotics, testing their effectiveness proved difficult due to several factors:

- Natural Remissions: Crohn's disease can cycle through flare ups and remissions, making it hard to determine if improvement is due to treatment or the disease's natural course.
- Placebo Effect: Short term improvements in clinical trials can be influenced by the placebo effect, which impacts up to 40% of patients.
- Diagnostic Challenges: Misdiagnosis is common, with up to 20% of Crohn's cases potentially being other diseases entirely.

Hope for the Future

Despite these hurdles, recent trials using macrolides like clarithromycin and rifabutin have shown promising results, especially with prolonged multi drug therapies lasting several years. As research progresses, these findings could shift the treatment paradigm for Crohn's disease, offering new hope for those who have struggled with ineffective treatments and invasive surgeries.

An Attempt at a Cure: RMAT Therapy for Crohn's Disease

In 1997, a groundbreaking trial in London tested a novel treatment for Crohn's disease, known as Rifabutin and Macrolide Antibiotic Therapy (RMAT). This approach combined rifabutin and clarithromycin, two antibiotics shown to have a synergistic effect against *Mycobacterium avium* subspecies *paratuberculosis* (MAP), the suspected bacterial trigger behind Crohn's disease.

The Results of the Initial Trial

The trial involved 52 patients with severe, treatment resistant Crohn's disease. Six patients had to discontinue due to intolerance to the antibiotics, although RMAT generally exhibited fewer side effects and better tolerance than standard immunosuppressive drugs. Among the remaining 46 patients, an astonishing 94% (43 patients) went into clinical remission after a year of treatment.

A two year follow up revealed that most patients remained symptom free without returning to their previous medications. Similar remission rates were observed in follow up trials at other research centers, reinforcing the initial findings.

Challenges in Achieving Long Term Remission

Despite the impressive remission rates, some patients relapsed after stopping treatment likely due to the difficulty in completely eradicating MAP or possible reinfection. Lead investigator Dr. John Hermon Taylor now recommends continuing RMAT for at least two years to maximize the chances of sustained remission. Like other chronic bacterial infections (e.g., leprosy), symptoms can temporarily worsen before improving.

Notably, RMAT not only alleviates symptoms but also promotes intestinal healing, a rare achievement in Crohn's treatments. As one researcher noted, "If this were cancer, we would be calling these long remissions a cure."

Barriers to Acceptance and Funding

Despite its success, RMAT trials faced significant hurdles:

- Funding Roadblocks: Hermon Taylor's grant proposals over 25 submissions worldwide were repeatedly rejected, and similar efforts by Dr. Rod Chiodini faced the same fate.
- Pharmaceutical Industry Resistance: The existing Crohn's treatment market, based on expensive, lifelong immunosuppressive drugs, generates billions for pharmaceutical companies. A potential cure threatens these profits, limiting corporate interest in supporting antibiotic based research.

The Push for Larger Trials
While early results are promising, larger, controlled trials are necessary to validate RMAT's effectiveness. A phase III clinical trial is underway in Australia, involving over 200 patients across seven major cities. The study is a double blind, multi center, controlled clinical trial the gold standard for medical research. Additionally, the National Institutes of Health (NIH) has reportedly initiated a controlled RMAT trial in the U.S.

Despite recruitment challenges, these trials could pave the way for a paradigm shift in Crohn's treatment, offering hope for long term remission and potentially a cure.

Milk, MAP, and Crohn's Disease: A Hidden Threat in Dairy Consumption

Dr. John Hermon Taylor, a leading expert in Crohn's disease and *Mycobacterium avium* subspecies *paratuberculosis* (MAP) genetics, has spent over two decades researching the link between MAP and Crohn's. He estimates that MAP could be responsible for 60% to 90% of all Crohn's cases, potentially accounting for the vast majority of instances worldwide.

Why Doesn't Everyone Get Crohn's Disease?

As with many infectious diseases, not everyone exposed to MAP develops Crohn's. This is similar to other bacterial infections:

- H. pylori infects roughly one third of Americans, yet only a fraction of those develop stomach ulcers.
- Only 1 in 300 people exposed to tuberculosis actually develop an active infection.

Genetic predisposition and environmental factors likely play significant roles in determining who develops Crohn's following MAP exposure.

The Milk Connection: How Are People Exposed to MAP?

The most common route of human exposure to MAP is through dairy consumption specifically, drinking milk from cows infected with Johne's disease (a MAP related illness in cattle). DNA fingerprinting has shown that all human MAP infections so far are of bovine origin, strongly implicating milk as the primary source. Cows with Johne's disease shed MAP bacteria in their milk, even when they appear healthy. Alarmingly, the bacteria may also be present inside pus cells found in milk. In the U.S., this issue is exacerbated by the country's relatively high legal limit for pus cell concentration in milk almost twice the international standard. Federal law permits over a drop of pus per glass of Grade A milk, raising concerns about facilitating the transmission of MAP.

Minimizing Exposure: A Public Health Concern
While more research is needed to confirm MAP's direct role in Crohn's disease, the association is strong enough that minimizing exposure should be a priority. Just as avoiding contact with tuberculosis patients can reduce infection risk, reducing consumption of milk from potentially infected cows or opting for pasteurized or plant based alternatives could help minimize exposure to MAP and, by extension, reduce the potential risk of Crohn's disease.

Pasteurization and MAP: Can Heat Treatments Prevent Crohn's Disease Risks?
Researchers in England tested milk straight from grocery store shelves for the presence of *Mycobacterium avium* subspecies *paratuberculosis* (MAP) DNA. The findings were concerning: up to 25% of milk cartons tested positive for MAP DNA, depending on the season. Interestingly, these seasonal spikes in MAP detection coincided with periods when Crohn's disease patients were more likely to experience relapses, hinting at a possible connection between consumption and disease flare ups.

The Pasteurization Problem: Does It Eliminate MAP?

Pasteurization was originally introduced to eliminate MAP's cousin, bovine tuberculosis (TB). The process involved heating milk to 62°C (144°F) for 30 minutes, effectively killing TB bacteria. Later, concerns about Q fever led to an increase in temperature to 63°C (145°F). Today's modern process, called High Temperature Short Time (HTST) pasteurization, heats milk to 72°C (162°F) for 15 seconds.

However, research has shown that MAP can survive much harsher conditions:

- Studies indicate that MAP can withstand 15 seconds at 90°C (194°F) far higher than standard pasteurization levels.
- MAP's survival is aided by its ability to hide in fat droplets, pus cells, and fecal clumps within milk, shielding it from heat exposure.

A Heat-Resistant Pathogen

MAP is now considered the second most heat resistant pathogen in the human food supply, surpassed only by prions (the infectious agents behind mad cow disease). This raises serious questions about whether current pasteurization methods are adequate to eliminate MAP from dairy products entirely.

What This Means for Public Health

The presence of MAP DNA in pasteurized milk doesn't necessarily mean the bacteria are alive detecting live MAP remains challenging due to the complexity of culturing it from milk. However, the potential survival of MAP through pasteurization could represent a hidden risk for consumers, particularly those genetically predisposed to Crohn's disease.

Given this uncertainty, researchers are calling for more stringent testing and possibly higher temperature pasteurization protocols. In the meantime, consumers concerned about MAP exposure can reduce their risk by choosing ultra pasteurized or plant based milk alternatives.

Johne's Disease on the Rise: A Growing Threat to Cattle and Human Health

According to the Food and Agriculture Organization (FAO) of the United Nations, Johne's disease is one of the most serious threats to the global cattle industry. Caused by *Mycobacterium avium* subspecies *paratuberculosis* (MAP), the disease affects cattle worldwide, but the United States is believed to have the highest prevalence of MAP infections globally.

The Scope of the Problem in the U.S.

A 1997 USDA report revealed alarming statistics: between 20% and 40% of U.S. dairy herds were infected with Johne's disease. However, the USDA acknowledged that this figure likely underestimates the true scope of the problem. Since milk from multiple herds is pooled together during transport and processing, the contamination risk extends far beyond infected herds, potentially affecting a significant portion of the U.S. milk supply.

A Link to Human Health?
The rising prevalence of Johne's disease in cattle appears to mirror the increasing rates of Crohn's disease in humans. With the U.S. also having the highest recorded incidence of Crohn's globally, some researchers believe this parallel isn't just a coincidence particularly given the potential link between MAP and Crohn's disease.

How Johne's Disease Spreads in Cattle
Johne's disease is primarily transmitted via the fecal oral route:
- Cows with chronic diarrhea contaminate their environment, increasing the likelihood of infecting other animals.
- A single infected cow can shed up to 100 trillion bacteria in a single day.
- Calves are particularly vulnerable, as ingesting even small amounts of contaminated manure can lead to infection.

The Role of Industrial Farming Practices
Modern farming practices exacerbate the spread of Johne's disease:
- Overcrowding cattle on increasingly smaller plots increases the risk of infection.
- Transporting animals between farms introduces MAP into new herds, facilitating rapid disease spread across regions.

Without significant changes to farming practices, experts warn that infection rates in dairy herds could eventually reach 100%. This would not only devastate the cattle industry but also raise serious concerns about the continued contamination of the milk supply and its potential connection to rising Crohn's disease cases in humans.

USDA Farce? Questionable Experiments and the MAP Controversy
As Johne's disease continues to spread among U.S. cattle herds, regulatory agencies like the USDA and FDA have faced mounting pressure to reassure the public that pasteurization effectively protects against *Mycobacterium avium* subspecies *paratuberculosis* (MAP). The official stance: 15 seconds at 72°C (162°F) the standard pasteurization protocol should eliminate any MAP present in milk.

The Scientific Evidence Against Pasteurization's Effectiveness
Despite government assurances, independent research has consistently shown that MAP can survive standard pasteurization. Many studies simulating real world conditions revealed that MAP survives the 15 second heat treatment, raising serious concerns about potential transmission through pasteurized milk.
Flawed USDA Experiment?
Critics argue that the USDA conducted a biased study designed to produce favorable results by weakening the bacteria beforehand:

- Weakened Bacteria: The USDA subjected MAP to starvation, high frequency sound waves, and freezing all methods known to weaken the bacterium's resilience.

- Methodological Errors: Allegations also include the use of inadequate culture media and a shortened observation period (only 2–3 months), while it typically takes 4 months or more for MAP to grow reliably in lab conditions.

As expected, the study concluded that no MAP bacteria survived pasteurization, leading to the USDA's controversial stance that pasteurized milk poses no risk of transmitting live MAP.

FDA's Questionable Endorsement
In 1998, the FDA followed the USDA's lead, dismissing previous research with a statement claiming that commercial pasteurization eliminates MAP risk. This decision ignored years of contradictory studies and scientific evidence pointing to the bacteria's survival through standard pasteurization processes.

The Reality of MAP Contamination in Milk
One major flaw in the USDA's defense is the assumption that MAP levels in milk are too low to pose a real threat. However:
- The true concentration of MAP in raw milk remains unknown.
- Cows infected with Johne's disease often suffer from chronic diarrhea, contaminating their udders with feces that may contain up to a trillion MAP bacteria per gram.
- During milking, bacteria from contaminated udders can easily enter the milk supply, potentially leading to widespread contamination when milk from multiple herds is pooled together.

Despite mounting scientific evidence, U.S. regulatory agencies continue to dismiss concerns about MAP survival in pasteurized milk. Critics argue that economic interests in the dairy industry may be influencing regulatory decisions, while public health risks remain inadequately addressed. Until more transparent and rigorous research is conducted, the debate over MAP's role in Crohn's disease and its survival through pasteurization will continue.

Off the Shelf: Live MAP Found in Pasteurized Milk

Despite growing evidence that standard pasteurization may not effectively eliminate *Mycobacterium avium* subspecies *paratuberculosis* (MAP) from milk, U.S. regulatory agencies and much of the agricultural press continue to cite the flawed USDA study, dismissing mounting scientific research to the contrary. Publications like *Hoard's Dairyman* echoed the USDA's conclusions, reassuring the public that "pasteurization destroys this dangerous disease." However, a year after the USDA study's publication, this assertion was definitively challenged by new research.

The Irish Study: Shattering the Illusion of Safety

In 1998, researchers conducted a groundbreaking study in Ireland, the European Union's leader in per capita milk consumption. They collected 31 cartons of commercially pasteurized milk from 16 retail outlets. The findings were alarming:

- 19% of the samples almost 1 in 5 cartons contained live MAP bacteria.

The results caused a national uproar in Ireland, sparking front page headlines and widespread public concern. Yet, despite the global attention, the issue received virtually no coverage in the United States, where the influence of the dairy industry and its extensive advertising campaigns (like the iconic "Got Milk?" ads) likely contributed to the media silence.

Dairy Industry Pushback and Media Silence
The Irish findings were described by crisis management experts as "enormous" and "horrific" in their implications for public health and the dairy industry's future. Industry leaders dismissed concerns and criticized researchers for not consulting them before publishing their findings. Meanwhile, dairy experts feared the news could accelerate the long term decline of milk consumption globally.

In the U.K., public pressure led the British government to launch a nationwide survey of 1,000 retail milk samples. Preliminary results, released in April 2000, revealed that 3% of milk cartons contained live MAP bacteria. To test positive, each quart of milk needed to contain at least one million MAP organisms a threshold with potentially serious health implications.

A Questionable Fix: Extended Pasteurization
In response to the initial concerns over MAP DNA detection, three major British supermarket chains Tesco, Sainsbury, and Safeway extended pasteurization times from 15 to 25 seconds in an attempt to reassure consumers. However, subsequent research revealed that even these extended times might be insufficient:

- Studies suggest MAP can survive exposure to pasteurization temperatures for up to 9 minutes or longer.

This raised doubts about whether any modest extension of pasteurization could fully eliminate MAP from milk.

The Ongoing Silence in the U.S.

Despite the growing body of international evidence, the American press and regulatory agencies have remained largely silent on the issue. Critics argue that powerful dairy industry lobbying and the economic importance of milk sales have stifled the conversation in the U.S., leaving consumers unaware of the potential health risks associated with contaminated dairy products.

The global scientific community continues to call for more stringent safety standards, improved pasteurization techniques, and increased transparency about the risks posed by MAP in dairy products an issue that remains under addressed in the United States.

Public Relations: Downplaying the MAP Risk

Despite mounting scientific evidence that Mycobacterium avium paratuberculosis (MAP) can survive pasteurization and potentially contribute to Crohn's disease, government officials and industry leaders have continued to downplay the threat. In the United Kingdom, following the discovery of live MAP in retail milk, the British Agriculture Minister publicly reassured citizens by stating, "I drink pasteurized milk and it is safe to do so... with confidence." This statement echoed similar false assurances made by officials during the mad cow disease (BSE) crisis a disease still estimated by the Royal Statistical Society to potentially claim up to 13 million lives among those unknowingly infected.

Echoes of Reassurance in the U.S.

Similar reassurances have been made in the United States. The USDA's National Animal Disease Center director expressed no hesitation in feeding pasteurized milk to his own child, insisting that the pasteurization process eliminated any potential health threats. The FDA has also continued to base its national milk safety policy on the flawed USDA study, despite international research proving the study's conclusions were inaccurate.

The U.S. employs the same pasteurization standards as Britain and Ireland, where live MAP bacteria have been consistently detected in pasteurized milk. Nonetheless, the FDA persists in claiming that pasteurization eliminates the risk of MAP infection contradicting growing scientific evidence.

Silencing the Doubts

The lack of transparency became apparent when Kurt Gutknecht, editor of the reputable *Wisconsin Agriculturist*, sought clarification from Joe Smucker, head of the FDA's Milk Safety Team. Smucker declined to comment, citing a lack of "clearance from the FDA." Even official spokespeople described this silence as "very unusual" behavior for the agency.

Repeated attempts to seek further answers from the FDA's Milk Safety Team were met with radio silence, raising concerns that the agency and industry insiders were actively suppressing discourse around the issue.

An Economic Time Bomb for the Dairy Industry

The dairy industry's reluctance to confront the MAP problem appears motivated by economic fears. If MAP were conclusively linked to human diseases like Crohn's, the financial implications for global dairy and animal agriculture industries could be catastrophic. An article in *Milk Science International* warned that any sensationalist handling of the data could trigger devastating repercussions for dairy producers worldwide.

Industry experts privately acknowledge the gravity of the situation, recognizing that the confirmation of MAP's role in human disease could fundamentally undermine public confidence in dairy safety resulting in massive economic fallout for both producers and regulatory bodies alike.

Hidden Threat: The Stealthy Spread of Johne's Disease

Johne's disease, caused by *Mycobacterium avium* subspecies *paratuberculosis* (MAP), is considered one of the most challenging diseases to detect and control within the cattle industry. Its resilience in the environment and ability to spread covertly through herds has earned it labels such as a "hidden threat" and an "insidious problem" for dairy farmers.

Why Is Johne's Disease So Hard to Detect?

One of the biggest challenges in managing Johne's disease is its long incubation period, which can range from 6 months to 15 years. Infection typically occurs during calfhood, but animals often show no clinical symptoms until adulthood. During this latent phase:

- Infected cows appear healthy but can still shed bacteria into the environment, unknowingly infecting other animals.
- This silent shedding allows the bacteria to spread extensively before the infection becomes apparent, embedding itself deeply in herds.

This phenomenon is known as the "iceberg effect" by the time one animal shows visible symptoms, there may be 5 to 20 others already infected in the herd. Worse, current diagnostic tests can only detect fewer than 30% of these hidden cases.

Clinical Challenges and Misdiagnosis
Even when clinical signs appear, Johne's disease is difficult to identify because:

- Symptoms such as progressive weight loss and decreased milk production are often mistaken for other conditions like malnutrition, intestinal parasites, or salmonellosis.
- Some infected animals go into remission periods, showing no symptoms for weeks or months.
- Farmers may cull underperforming cows without requesting veterinary testing, allowing the disease to spread unnoticed.

Why Traditional Control Methods Fail
Efforts to manage Johne's disease through traditional measures, like culling infected animals, have largely

failed due to the disease's covert progression and environmental persistence:

- The bacteria can survive outside the host for extended periods, contaminating soil, water, and pastures.
- Even if visibly infected animals are removed, the underlying infection remains entrenched within the herd.

Extreme proposals, like complete herd disposal and disinfecting pastures, are considered economically infeasible due to the widespread nature of the infection.

Preventing Transmission: Segregation and Hygiene
The next best approach to control Johne's disease focuses on segregation and strict hygiene:

- Infected animals should be isolated from the rest of the herd.
- Boot washing, udder cleaning, and other hygiene protocols are crucial to prevent the spread of infection through manure.
- Surveys reveal compliance issues, with about one third of farms failing to wash cows' udders before collecting colostrum or milking practices that increase the risk of contamination.

Calf Management and Animal Welfare Concerns
Because some calves are infected in utero, immediate separation from their mothers after birth is recommended to reduce infection risk:

- Currently, two thirds of U.S. dairy operations separate calves within 24 hours of birth.

- Animal welfare advocates criticize this practice, viewing it as harmful to calf mother bonding and potentially unnecessary in many cases.

The Problem of Waste Management
Disposing of feces from infected cattle presents another challenge:
- Some experts suggest using specialized landfills to prevent environmental contamination.
- Others have proposed the hazardous idea of spreading infected manure on permanent cropland, which could further facilitate the spread of MAP to new areas and populations.

The Bigger Picture: A Threat to Public Health?
Given the increasing evidence linking MAP to Crohn's disease in humans, the covert spread of Johne's disease in cattle poses not just an economic and animal welfare issue but also a potential public health crisis. Without stricter control measures and improved testing, Johne's disease may continue to silently proliferate both in cattle herds and possibly in the human population through contaminated dairy products.

Conspiracy of Silence: The Hidden Crisis of Johne's Disease in the Dairy Industry
Despite its devastating effects on milk production and its ability to decimate entire herds, Johne's disease remains a taboo subject in the dairy industry. Instead of open discussions about the disease, there is a persistent "conspiracy of silence" that suppresses

dialogue, obstructs research, and keeps both farmers and consumers largely unaware of the scope of the issue.

A Whispered Secret Among Farmers
Within farming communities, Johne's disease is often treated as a shameful secret:

- Farmers discuss the disease in hushed tones, fearing stigma and financial repercussions.
- One dairy scientist noted that in decades of experience, he had never witnessed an open discussion about Johne's disease, highlighting the depth of the secrecy.
- A farmer candidly compared the stigma surrounding Johne's disease to AIDS, calling it "a dirty word" that no one dares to mention.

This climate of fear leads many farmers to hide outbreaks of the disease in their herds, avoiding acknowledgment or action to prevent financial loss, public scrutiny, or damage to their farm's reputation.

Industry Wide Silence and Suppression
The secrecy surrounding Johne's disease extends beyond individual farmers to the entire dairy industry:

- According to the *Journal of Dairy Science*, fear of negative consumer reactions stifles open scientific discussions about Johne's disease.
- Researcher Dr. Rod Chiodini has argued that the dairy industry's primary concern is not public health but the potential for "bad press" that could damage profits and consumer trust.

This deliberate suppression of information creates an environment where scientific research is discouraged, and the real risks of Johne's disease especially its potential link to Crohn's disease remain underexplored.

A Widespread Lack of Awareness
The consequences of this silence are stark:

- A USDA national survey revealed that nearly 50% of dairy farmers had no knowledge of Johne's disease, despite its widespread prevalence.
- Alarmingly, farmers with the largest herds which are at the greatest risk of infection were the least informed about the disease.

Karen Meyer, former Executive Director of the Paratuberculosis Awareness and Research Association (PARA), placed the blame squarely on industry representatives who, she argued, had failed to properly educate and protect farmers. Speaking at a USDA meeting, she challenged dairy producers to confront the issue head on and criticized industry leaders for their lack of proactive engagement.

The Moral Responsibility of Farmers
Many advocates believe that farmers would take action if they fully understood the potential public health implications of Johne's disease:

- Meyer told the *Wisconsin Agriculturist* that most farmers "would be heartbroken" if they knew their practices could contribute to making consumers sick.
- She emphasized that providing accurate information to farmers could help break the cycle of ignorance, stigma, and silence that perpetuates the spread of the disease.

A Call for Transparency and Action
The ongoing silence around Johne's disease not only endangers cattle and threatens the sustainability of dairy farming but may also have serious implications for human health. Breaking this silence requires:

- Open scientific discussion without fear of damaging the dairy industry's reputation.
- Improved education and awareness among farmers, particularly those managing large herds.
- Transparent communication with the public about the potential risks associated with Johne's disease.

Until the industry faces these realities openly, Johne's disease will continue to spread in the shadows, posing a hidden threat to both animal and human health.

US Inaction: A Failure to Address the Growing Threat of Johne's Disease

Despite the growing evidence linking Johne's disease and its causative agent, *Mycobacterium avium* subspecies *paratuberculosis* (MAP), to Crohn's disease and the severe economic impact on the cattle industry, the USDA has been accused of neglecting the issue. Critics argue that the government continues to "bury its head in the sand," underfunding research and failing to implement meaningful control measures.

Underfunded and Underregulated

The USDA allocates less than 1% of its animal disease grant budget to research on Johne's disease. As Alan Kennedy, co-founder of the Paratuberculosis Awareness and Research Association (PARA) and a Crohn's sufferer, put it, this reflects a conflict of interest. The USDA's dual mandate to both regulate food safety and promote agricultural products creates a situation ripe for regulatory inaction.

Despite identifying the first U.S. case of Johne's in 1908, no mandatory control program exists, even though scientists have warned about the disease's dangers since 1922. Today, USDA estimates suggest that up to 750,000 cattle in the U.S. are infected with MAP a number that continues to grow due to a lack of effective containment measures.

Why the Disease Is Spreading Unchecked
The unchecked spread of Johne's disease is largely due to the absence of movement restrictions on infected animals:

- Asymptomatic carriers often introduce the disease into new herds since infected cows can appear healthy at the time of sale.
- Studies reveal that infected herds are just as likely as non infected herds to sell replacement cows to other farms.

While regulatory veterinarians acknowledge that restricting the movement of infected animals is essential, such measures have been resisted due to pressure from the livestock industry. In fact, changes to the Code of Federal Regulations have recently removed restrictions on the interstate transport of Johne's positive animals, undermining disease control efforts.

Voluntary Programs: A Recipe for Failure
Efforts to control Johne's disease in the U.S. rely largely on voluntary programs:

- The National Johne's Working Group, formed in 1994, remains composed primarily of industry representatives, including officials from the National Milk Producers Federation and the National Cattlemen's Beef Association.
- Instead of mandating testing or movement restrictions, the group has opposed making Johne's a reportable disease and has resisted any compulsory regulations.

Predictably, these voluntary measures have failed:

- Only 1% of dairy operations have joined the national paratuberculosis certification program.
- Fewer than 15% of dairy producers test for Johne's disease regularly, citing the high costs associated with testing.

International Progress Highlights U.S. Inaction
While the U.S. lags behind, other countries have taken decisive action:

- The Netherlands has pledged to eradicate paratuberculosis through a compulsory eradication program, citing human health risks.
- Sweden has made significant progress through mandatory control measures.
- Australia is actively certifying herds with an eye toward eventual eradication.

In contrast, the U.S. risks falling behind in global dairy markets, potentially jeopardizing its $700 million dairy export industry if international trade restrictions are introduced due to the country's inadequate response to Johne's disease.

Industry Resistance and Suppression of Dialogue
Attempts to address Johne's disease in the U.S. are often met with industry resistance:

- Researchers and veterinarians who speak out are frequently marginalized, with no recognition or support from the dairy industry.
- Christine Rossiter of Cornell University notes that those who attempt to tackle Johne's disease face professional risks and lack industry backing.
-

At an international conference, Dr. Rod Chiodini warned that the dairy industry's continued silence could mirror the fate of the tobacco industry, facing accusations of a cover up and potentially severe legal liabilities.

A Brewing Public Health Scandal?
Legal experts like Paul Strandberg, Assistant Attorney General of Minnesota, have cautioned that the dairy industry's reluctance to address the MAP Crohn's disease link could spark major public backlash. If the connection becomes widely acknowledged, the industry could face investigations, lawsuits, and media scrutiny akin to the mad cow disease crisis in Europe.

Until the USDA and dairy industry take decisive action including mandatory testing, movement restrictions, and adequate funding for research the U.S. will remain vulnerable to both economic and public health consequences from the silent spread of Johne's disease.

Off the Shelf USA: The Fight to Test U.S. Milk for MAP
Despite mounting global evidence linking *Mycobacterium avium* subspecies *paratuberculosis* (MAP) to Crohn's disease and its survival in pasteurized milk, efforts to investigate the presence of live MAP in U.S. retail milk supplies have been systematically blocked. Leading experts and advocacy groups, particularly the Paratuberculosis Awareness and Research Association (PARA), have long called for government funded studies to determine the extent of MAP contamination in American dairy products.
Industry Resistance to Testing

Prominent researchers like Dr. Rod Chiodini and Dr. John Hermon Taylor, both recognized authorities on MAP and its possible role in Crohn's disease, have submitted repeated proposals to the USDA and FDA to conduct retail milk testing. Year after year, these proposals have been rejected a refusal that many believe reflects pressure from the powerful dairy industry rather than sound scientific reasoning.

At a U.S. Animal Health Association (USAHA) meeting, a resolution proposing retail milk testing for MAP was voted down. John Adams, a representative of the National Milk Producers Federation and a member of the Johne's Disease Working Group, opposed the motion, stating:

"The FDA has already stated their position. They are confident that pasteurized milk is safe. We don't need to test retail milk."

In response, Steve Merkel, a PARA co-founder whose wife had suffered from Crohn's disease since 1960, countered with a pointed question:

"If milk is as safe as you say it is, then retail testing will simply confirm that fact. Are you afraid of what you might find?"

Nevertheless, the resolution was overwhelmingly rejected by the assembly.

Behind Closed Doors: Blocking the Science

In 1999, PARA successfully pushed two resolutions through the Johne's Disease Committee:

1. Testing of retail milk and dairy products for live MAP bacteria.
2. Research to determine cooking temperatures required to kill MAP in ground beef.

While these resolutions were unanimously passed in open committee, they were quietly overturned behind closed doors a move PARA viewed as a deliberate attempt by the USAHA to maintain ignorance about MAP contamination in food products.

Justifications for Inaction: A Conflict of Interest?

The USAHA justified blocking the resolutions by citing doubts about MAP's role in Crohn's disease, stating:

"There was much concern about the feasibility of end product testing of milk and meat for an organism that science has not confirmed as being the cause of Crohn's in humans."

In a letter to the USAHA president elect, PARA sharply criticized this rationale, calling it "self serving" and "contemptuous" of both the dairy industry's own members and the American public. PARA accused the organization of deliberately choosing to remain part of the problem rather than seeking a solution.

What's at Stake?

Advocates argue that retail milk testing would either:

- Confirm the safety of pasteurized milk, or
- Reveal contamination, prompting much needed reforms to protect public health.

Either outcome would provide clarity. However, critics argue that the dairy industry's resistance stems from fear of economic fallout if contamination were proven echoing concerns similar to those raised during the mad cow disease crisis and drawing uncomfortable parallels with the tobacco industry's historical suppression of health risks.

Until comprehensive testing is conducted, the U.S. remains vulnerable to the potential health consequences of MAP contamination, while public awareness of this hidden risk remains dangerously low.

Gambling with Lives: The Dairy Industry's Risky Bet on Johne's Disease

The stance taken by the U.S. Animal Health Association (USAHA) and the broader American dairy industry reflects a dangerous gamble one that prioritizes short term financial stability over long term public health concerns. Similar to the disastrous mismanagement of mad cow disease (BSE) in Britain, U.S. dairy authorities appear willing to defer action on paratuberculosis (*Mycobacterium avium* subspecies *paratuberculosis*, or MAP) until conclusive proof emerges of its link to Crohn's disease.

Echoes of the Mad Cow Crisis

In Britain, beef industry leaders initially dismissed concerns about mad cow disease, describing it as "something that bears watching" but not warranting immediate action until a definitive connection to human health risks was established. This strategy, however, backfired spectacularly:

- The delayed response led to a public health disaster and eroded consumer trust.
- Social science studies suggest that the government's repeated assurances of beef safety caused the most lasting damage to public confidence.

The American dairy industry now risks following the same path, gambling with the health of millions by choosing inaction despite mounting scientific evidence of MAP's potential link to Crohn's disease.

The Economic Gamble

The financial stakes for the U.S. livestock industry are already high:

- Johne's disease costs the American livestock sector over $1 billion annually due to lost productivity, reduced milk yields, and herd culling.

- A collapse in consumer confidence if the connection between MAP and Crohn's disease is proven could lead to even greater financial devastation.

Industry's Lip Service or Genuine Concern?

Experts like Dr. Rod Chiodini argue that, for now, the dairy industry's response is largely "lip service" an attempt to maintain a public image of concern while avoiding any meaningful action. This strategy serves to:

- Project an image of responsibility without implementing significant changes.
- Avoid costly interventions that might disrupt the industry's profits.

However, as the Paratuberculosis Awareness and Research Association (PARA) warned in an open letter:

"If dairy products become associated with the dreadful, life destroying disease known as Crohn's disease, your markets may also collapse and may never recover."

The Risk to Public Trust

The dairy industry has spent decades carefully cultivating the image of milk as an essential part of good nutrition. If MAP is definitively linked to Crohn's disease, that image could be irreparably damaged. Consumers would likely lose trust not just in dairy products but also in the regulatory agencies tasked with protecting public health.

A Cautionary Conclusion Inaction may seem like the path of least resistance for the dairy industry today, but the long-term consequences could be catastrophic:

- Public health risks will continue to grow as Johne's disease spreads unchecked in cattle herds.
- Economic fallout could mirror, or even surpass, the consequences of Britain's mad cow disaster.

The industry now faces a choice: act proactively to address the risks posed by MAP, or continue gambling with both consumer health and the future of dairy markets a bet that history suggests they are unlikely to win.

Other Dairy Products: The Hidden Risks Beyond Milk

While much of the concern surrounding *Mycobacterium avium* subspecies *paratuberculosis* (MAP) has focused on milk, other dairy products may also serve as potential carriers of this resilient bacterium. Experts argue that focusing solely on milk testing ignores the broader risk posed by a variety of common dairy products consumed across the United States.

The Cheese Concern: A Hidden Reservoir of MAP?

A significant risk comes from cheese, especially since one third of cheese produced in the U.S. is made from raw, unpasteurized milk:

- Raw milk cheeses likely harbor the highest concentrations of MAP bacteria.
- Cheese manufacturers typically rely on the product's salty, acidic environment to inhibit bacterial growth. However, studies have shown that MAP can withstand these conditions far better than many other bacteria.

- Even less robust mycobacteria have been found to survive in soft cheeses for at least 3 months and in hard cheeses for up to 10 months.

At the University of Wisconsin, researchers are currently investigating MAP's ability to survive in various cheese products an effort that could shed light on whether cheese consumption poses a significant public health risk.

Ice Cream: A Cold Survival Strategy

Freezing, commonly used in the preservation of dairy products like ice cream, offers no guarantee of eliminating MAP:

- Research has demonstrated that MAP can survive freezing for at least a year.
- Ice cream may also be produced using less rigorously pasteurized milk, further increasing the likelihood that live MAP bacteria could survive the manufacturing process.

Given how widely consumed ice cream is across all age groups, including vulnerable populations such as children, the potential risk warrants urgent investigation.

Other Dairy Products: An Overlooked Threat

The potential for MAP contamination extends to a wide range of dairy products:

- Butter: Since MAP can survive in high fat environments, butter could serve as another vector for the bacteria.
- Yogurt: Despite its probiotic nature, the fermentation process used in yogurt production does not guarantee the elimination of MAP.
- Infant formula: Arguably the most concerning, as infants represent a highly vulnerable population. If MAP contamination occurs in infant formula

derived from infected milk, it could have long term health implications.

The Need for Comprehensive Testing

Given MAP's resilience across various environments including high salt concentrations, acidity, and freezing temperatures researchers and public health advocates are calling for comprehensive testing across all dairy products, not just milk. These products must be scrutinized to determine whether current production standards are sufficient to eliminate MAP contamination and reduce the potential public health risks associated with Crohn's disease.

Until such testing is conducted, consumers remain unaware of the potential risks lurking in their everyday dairy products, and regulatory agencies continue to overlook a potentially significant threat to public health.

Beef: An Overlooked Source of MAP Contamination?

While much of the concern surrounding *Mycobacterium avium* subspecies *paratuberculosis* (MAP) has focused on milk and dairy products, evidence suggests that beef could also be a significant source of contamination. Standard veterinary protocols recommend that cows diagnosed with Johne's disease be sent to slaughter yet there are no regulations preventing the sale of beef from infected animals for human consumption since MAP is not officially recognized as a human pathogen.

Infected Meat in the Food Supply

Infected cows, particularly those in the end stages of Johne's disease, may carry trillions of MAP bacteria:

- These animals, often severely emaciated and suffering from advanced disease, are frequently processed into ground beef.
- Advocates for Crohn's disease patients have described the inclusion of infected meat in the human food supply as "abhorrent" and "nauseating."

Even if muscle tissue from infected cows is initially free of MAP, the slaughtering process increases the risk of contamination:

- Advanced Johne's disease causes MAP bacteria to circulate through the bloodstream, potentially infecting internal organs and muscle tissue.
- Fecal contamination during processing is a serious concern, as evidenced by recurring E. coli outbreaks linked to meat products.

How Prevalent Is Johne's Disease in Beef Cattle?

While dairy cows are most commonly associated with Johne's disease, the beef industry is not immune:

- In 1984, around 1% of U.S. beef cattle tested positive for Johne's disease.
- Due to the disease's hidden nature and the absence of a mandatory reporting system, the actual prevalence today could be significantly higher.

Awareness among beef producers remains shockingly low:

- A USDA report revealed that nearly 70% of U.S. beef producers had never heard of Johne's disease.
- Fewer than 10% had any knowledge of the disease beyond simple name recognition.

Cooking May Not Eliminate the Risk

Even standard cooking practices might not effectively kill MAP bacteria:

- MAP is considered the most heat resistant mycobacterium found in retail beef.
- While the USDA recommends cooking hamburgers to an internal temperature of 71°C (160°F) and roasts or steaks to 63°C (145°F), studies suggest that prolonged exposure to temperatures of at least 74°C (165°F) may be necessary to eliminate MAP completely.
- MAP also resists nitrites and smoking processes, meaning it could survive in processed meats like sausages.

Beyond Beef: Other Meat Products at Risk

While cattle remain the primary concern, MAP contamination could extend to other meats:

- Pigs and chickens have shown susceptibility to paratuberculosis, although further research is needed to confirm transmission pathways to humans.

Milk vs. Meat: Which Is More Dangerous?

Interestingly, milk may pose a greater risk for transmitting MAP than meat:

- Milk's natural buffering properties protect MAP from the acidic environment of the stomach, potentially allowing the bacteria to reach the intestines.
- In contrast, MAP's ability to survive the digestive process from meat consumption is less certain, though still concerning.

The Need for Regulatory Action

Despite these risks, there are still no mandatory controls in place for MAP infected beef in the U.S. Without clear action, including stricter testing protocols and mandatory disease reporting, consumers may continue to unknowingly consume potentially contaminated meat, leaving public health vulnerable to a largely ignored threat.

Water: An Overlooked Vector for MAP Contamination
While much of the concern around *Mycobacterium avium* subspecies *paratuberculosis* (MAP) has focused on dairy and meat products, water supplies may also serve as a hidden transmission route for this resilient bacterium. Contaminated surface waters especially those exposed to agricultural runoff pose a potential risk to many communities across the United States.

MAP: A Resilient Environmental "Superbug"
MAP has earned the nickname "superbug" due to its extraordinary ability to survive in harsh environmental conditions:

- It has existed on Earth for over a billion years, evolving adaptations that allow it to persist in various ecosystems.
- Its thick, waxy cell wall makes it particularly resistant to degradation and environmental stress.

Research shows that MAP can survive for extended periods:

- 9 months in mud
- Nearly 1 year in manure
- Up to 2 years in water supplies

Agricultural Runoff: A Major Contamination Source
Agricultural practices, particularly in regions with intensive cattle farming, contribute significantly to MAP contamination in water systems:

- Runoff from infected cattle manure can leach into rivers, lakes, and other bodies of water.
- Many municipal water supplies draw from these contaminated surface waters, raising concerns about public exposure.

Water Treatment: Are Current Methods Effective?

Standard domestic water treatment processes such as filtration and chlorination are likely ineffective against MAP:

- The bacterium's waxy outer layer shields it from chemical disinfectants like chlorine.
- Conventional filtration systems may not be equipped to trap such small, resilient organisms effectively.

This means that even treated municipal water supplies could still harbor live MAP bacteria, posing an unrecognized public health risk.

Global Evidence of Contamination

Several studies have raised alarms about MAP contamination in drinking water:

- European studies have successfully cultured live MAP bacteria from drinking water supplies, prompting further investigations into the safety of municipal water.
- A study in a major American city also detected MAP in the water supply, though this finding received little public attention.

In response, Europe's Drinking Water Inspectorate has launched a formal investigation into the distribution and persistence of MAP during water treatment processes. Despite similar risks in the U.S., no comparable national inquiry has been initiated.

The Need for Proactive Measures in the U.S.

Given MAP's potential to survive in water systems and its suspected link to Crohn's disease, researchers and public health advocates are calling for:

- Comprehensive testing of municipal water supplies for MAP contamination.
- Upgraded water treatment methods that specifically target resistant bacteria like MAP.
- Increased monitoring of agricultural runoff to prevent further contamination of surface waters.

Until these steps are taken, millions of Americans may unknowingly be exposed to MAP through their tap water, underscoring the urgent need for greater regulatory oversight and scientific investigation into this underappreciated transmission route.

2000: A Groundbreaking Discovery Linking Breast Milk and MAP

In April 2000, a pivotal study published in the *American Journal of Gastroenterology* revealed findings with profound implications for understanding the potential transmission of Mycobacterium avium subspecies paratuberculosis (MAP) and its possible role in Crohn's disease.

MAP Detected in Human Breast Milk

Researchers, aware that cows with Johne's disease shed MAP bacteria into their milk, began to investigate whether a similar phenomenon could occur in humans specifically, whether mothers with Crohn's disease might also shed MAP in their breast milk. Their hypothesis was further supported by previous reports of women with other mycobacterial diseases (such as leprosy) transmitting bacteria through breast milk.

The study examined two mothers with Crohn's disease who had recently given birth:

- MAP bacteria were found growing in the breast milk of both mothers.
- No MAP was detected in breast milk samples from healthy control mothers without Crohn's disease.

What This Means for Crohn's Disease Transmission

While breastfeeding has not been identified as a risk factor for Crohn's disease and may even provide protective health benefits this discovery raises important questions:

- It offers further support for the theory that MAP may play a role in the development of Crohn's disease.
- It suggests a potential new transmission route for MAP from mother to child, which could expose new generations to the bacterium early in life.

Long Term Implications for Public Health

This finding has significant ramifications:

- It highlights the need for further research to understand whether MAP transmission through breastfeeding could contribute to the onset of Crohn's disease later in life.
- It underscores the importance of studying MAP's role in early childhood exposure and its potential impact on the immune system.

The Need for Further Research

Although the study's sample size was small, the presence of MAP in the breast milk of mothers with Crohn's disease underscores the urgency for more comprehensive research:

- Larger studies are needed to determine whether MAP transmission through breastfeeding is a widespread phenomenon.

- Investigations into possible preventative measures should be prioritized for mothers with Crohn's disease to minimize potential risks of early life MAP exposure.

This discovery deepens the scientific understanding of how MAP may influence the development of Crohn's disease and raises critical questions about protecting future generations from potential exposure.

Recommendations for Action: Addressing the MAP Crisis in the U.S.

Despite overwhelming evidence that *Mycobacterium avium* subspecies *paratuberculosis* (MAP) is a potential human pathogen, it continues to be tolerated in the U.S. food supply. In stark contrast, other countries such as Ireland have taken decisive action to protect public health by implementing strict regulations that remove MAP infected cattle from the food chain.

Ireland's Proactive Response: A Model for the U.S.

Following the discovery of live MAP bacteria in retail milk, the Food Safety Authority of Ireland introduced aggressive measures:

- Cattle infected with Johne's disease are now excluded from both the meat and dairy supply.
- The meat of infected cows is no longer considered fit for human consumption.
- Milk from infected cows is dumped rather than processed and sold.

Karen Meyer of the Paratuberculosis Awareness and Research Association (PARA) praised Ireland's response, stating:

"The government of Ireland is to be commended for exercising the precautionary principle. Instead of trying to sweep the problem under the rug, they acted swiftly to give human health priority over special interests."

The U.S. Problem: A Crisis Exponentially Worse

While Ireland has only 12 reported cases of Johne's disease among its 7.6 million cattle, the U.S. prevalence is estimated to be 20,000 times higher:

- Despite having the highest prevalence of Johne's disease in the world, the U.S. has taken no mandatory action.
- The National Johne's Working Group continues to recommend only voluntary measures focused on cattle health, leaving human health unprotected.

Concrete Steps for Immediate Action

Experts argue that several actions could have an immediate impact:

1. Remove Clinically Infected Cattle from the Food Supply
   Modeling suggests that eliminating meat and milk from visibly infected animals could significantly reduce public exposure. According to experts, it would take just six months to clean up America's herds if milk from Johne's positive cows were banned from sale.

2. Make Crohn's Disease a Reportable Illness
   Mandating that Crohn's disease cases be officially recorded would help monitor potential links between MAP exposure and human health, increasing scientific understanding of the disease's spread.

3. Challenge the FDA's Outdated Position on Pasteurization
   The FDA's official stance that standard pasteurization effectively eliminates MAP is no

longer scientifically valid. Studies in Britain and Ireland have demonstrated that MAP can survive standard pasteurization processes and remain viable in the food supply.

4. Demand Transparency Through the Freedom of Information Act

An extensive Freedom of Information Act (FOIA) investigation could uncover documents suppressed by government agencies. For example, a Canadian risk assessment linking MAP to Crohn's disease was classified as "Protected. Not for Distribution" and never publicly released.

A Call for the Precautionary Principle in U.S. Policy

Experts like Dr. John Hermon Taylor warn of a potential public health disaster:

"There is overwhelming evidence that we are sitting on a public health disaster of tragic proportions."

In Europe, the precautionary principle which dictates that preventive action should be taken when reasonable suspicion of harm exists guides health and environmental policy. The principle suggests:

"If one has a reasonable suspicion that something bad might happen, one has an obligation to try to stop it."

Avoiding a Public Health Catastrophe

The consequences of inaction are clear. Lessons from the mad cow disease crisis in Britain reveal the dangers of delaying action until definitive proof is established:

- A British inquiry concluded that a "lack of proof" led to a disaster that might have been prevented with more proactive measures.
- Millions of lives could have been saved if the government had acted sooner, based on the

precautionary principle rather than waiting for irrefutable evidence.

The Path Forward for the U.S.

Given the scale of the Johne's disease problem in the U.S., policymakers must:

- Enact mandatory testing and removal of infected cattle from the food supply.
- Implement stricter controls over dairy and meat processing.
- Prioritize transparency and consumer protection over industry profits.

Failing to act now risks not only the public's health but also the long term stability of the U.S. dairy and beef industries. An ounce of prevention today could save millions of lives tomorrow.

On a Personal Level: Reducing Your Risk of MAP Exposure

For individuals concerned about the potential health risks posed by *Mycobacterium avium* subspecies *paratuberculosis* (MAP) especially those with Crohn's disease or a genetic predisposition advocacy groups like Action Research and the Paratuberculosis Awareness and Research Association (PARA) offer practical recommendations to minimize exposure.

How to Reduce Your Risk: Boiling Dairy Products

The most effective method to eliminate live MAP bacteria from dairy products is high heat treatment:

- Boiling dairy products (heating to 100°C or 212°F) can effectively sterilize milk, cheese, yogurt, and butter.
- For cheese, grilling until it bubbles or baking in oven cooked meals like lasagna is

recommended to ensure the product reaches sufficient temperatures to kill MAP bacteria.

- Similar heat treatments should be applied to yogurt, butter, and other dairy derivatives.

Why Isn't Milk Pasteurized at Higher Temperatures?

The dairy industry resists raising pasteurization temperatures because of potential changes in the taste of milk:

- The Irish Food Safety Authority acknowledges that heating milk beyond a certain threshold causes unacceptable taste changes.
- Steve Merkel of PARA argues that taste should take a backseat to health concerns:

"Even if milk doesn't taste the same as it did, human health must take precedence over taste."

The Hidden Risk: Even Dead MAP May Be Harmful

While stricter pasteurization can kill MAP bacteria, recent research suggests that even dead MAP organisms may still trigger harmful immune responses:

- The MAP vaccine made from killed bacteria can cause severe and chronic inflammation in humans if accidentally injected, sometimes requiring amputation due to the body's extreme immune reaction.
- Similar immune reactions have been observed with closely related bacteria, such as those responsible for leprosy.

This raises concerns that even pasteurized milk, though free of live bacteria, could still contain remnants of MAP proteins that might stimulate inflammation in susceptible individuals.

The Safer Option: Avoid Dairy Products Altogether

Given these uncertainties, avoiding dairy products entirely may be the safest course of action:

- The exact infectious dose of MAP for humans is unknown.
- The true extent of milk contamination in the U.S. has not been adequately studied or disclosed.

Dr. Benjamin Spock, one of the most influential pediatricians of all time, advocated for a vegan diet for children, citing multiple health reasons now potentially including the risk of MAP exposure.

Plant Based Alternatives: A Healthy, Risk Free Solution

Fortunately, avoiding dairy does not mean sacrificing taste or nutrition. There are numerous plant based alternatives available:

- Soy, almond, rice, and oat milks offer similar textures and nutritional profiles to traditional cow's milk.
- Non dairy cheeses, ice creams, and yogurts are widely available and often fortified with calcium and vitamin D.

For those at risk of Crohn's disease or simply looking to minimize potential MAP exposure, transitioning to plant based alternatives may offer a safer, healthier path forward.

A Call to Confront the Hidden Crisis of Johne's Disease, the ongoing epidemic of Johne's disease, much like the past crisis of mad cow disease, stands as a stark indictment of factory farming and the industrialization of animal agriculture. Intensive confinement systems where animals are raised in unnatural, overcrowded conditions pose not only a threat to the global environment but also to public health.

Factory Farming and Global Health Risks

The concentration of animals raised for food production has historically led to devastating consequences:

- The 1918 influenza pandemic, the deadliest epidemic in recorded history, claimed the lives of over 40 million people. Researchers now believe that the virus likely emerged due to the unnatural density and close proximity of pigs and ducks raised for slaughter.
- Today, similar risks are being repeated with diseases like Johne's disease, which continues to spread due to the intensive farming practices still dominating the livestock industry.

An Industry and Government Failing Public Health

This growing crisis not only reflects the dangers of modern farming but also reveals the troubling complicity of an industry and a government that seems more committed to protecting corporate interests than safeguarding public health:

- Despite mounting evidence linking Mycobacterium avium subspecies paratuberculosis (MAP) to Crohn's disease, both the dairy industry and government agencies have largely resisted implementing effective control measures.
- As Karen Meyer of the Paratuberculosis Awareness and Research Association (PARA) aptly told the *LA Times*:

"There comes a point in time where consumer health takes precedence over commercial concerns."

The Human Cost of Inaction

Every few hours in the U.S., another child is diagnosed with Crohn's disease, potentially condemning them to a lifetime of chronic pain, hospitalization, and suffering:

- A growing body of research strongly suggests a causative link between MAP and Crohn's disease.
- Yet this pressing public health issue remains largely ignored by the dairy industry, relegated to the background as an inconvenient concern.

The Need for Consumer Action

The consumer movement must take the lead where government and industry have failed:

- Raise awareness about the potential health risks associated with dairy consumption and the role of MAP in Crohn's disease.
- Demand transparency, testing, and the removal of infected animals from the food supply.
- Support policies and advocacy efforts aimed at making Crohn's disease a reportable illness and pushing for stricter regulations on the dairy and meat industries.

Turning Up the Heat on Industry Inaction

It's time to move this issue from the back burner to the forefront of public health policy. Consumer pressure has driven significant change in industries before, and it can do so again:

- By demanding stricter safety standards and prioritizing human health over corporate profit, consumers can help prevent what could become a public health disaster.
- Inaction now could lead to consequences that mirror past health crises, but decisive action today could safeguard future generations from the devastating impact of this hidden epidemic.

The hidden crisis of foodborne illness in the U.S., particularly the potential link between Mycobacterium avium paratuberculosis (MAP) and Crohn's disease, lays bare a chilling truth: our health is too often sacrificed for profit. This chapter has peeled back the veil on a system that buries inconvenient evidence studies showing MAP in dairy and water, whistleblower accounts of regulatory inaction, and the stark absence of food safety reforms that could prevent chronic diseases. For Crohn's patients like me, the discovery that our suffering might stem from pathogens in everyday food is both infuriating and empowering. The $13 billion inflammatory bowel disease market thrives on our dependency, with biologics costing $20,000 $85,000 annually while affordable antibiotic therapies, inspired by pioneers like Rod Chiodini and Thomas Borody, languish in obscurity. This is no accident; it's a calculated silence, driven by agribusiness interests and a medical establishment resistant to paradigms that threaten revenue. As I reflect on my journey, I see the echoes of this conspiracy in every flare, every bill, every dismissed question about MAP. Yet, the Crohn's community is not powerless. We must demand action: mandatory MAP testing in food supplies, funding for anti-MAP trials, and transparency in regulatory decisions. Project Censored's spirit reminds us that truth, though buried, can be unearthed through collective resolve. We stand unbowed, unbroken, and ready to expose this hidden epidemic, fighting for a future where our plates don't poison us and our diseases aren't profited from. Let this be our rallying cry: no more silence, no more suffering only answers and accountability.

Afterword

Bayer's Sinister Legacy

In the shadowed corridors of history, a tale of unspeakable audacity emerges one that stains the name of Bayer, a pharmaceutical giant born in Germany's industrial heartland. In the early 1940s, as the Holocaust's machinery ground millions into dust, Bayer dispatched a letter to the Nazi regime, its tone as clinical as it was chilling: "Send us 150 Jewish women for experimental testing." The Nazis, ever eager to oblige their corporate allies, plucked 150 healthy women from the camps women not frail or infirm, but robust, their vitality a stark contrast to the fate awaiting them. Within three months, all 150 lay dead, their bodies a silent testament to Bayer's pursuits. Undaunted, the company penned a second missive: "The results are a resounding success. We require another 150 subjects." Another shipment arrived, and they too perished 300 healthy lives extinguished in half a year. Success, Bayer proclaimed, though the graves offered no applause. What were they crafting in those blood-soaked labs? The letters, preserved in archives, boast of triumph, yet the purpose remains a sinister enigma drug, perhaps, or something more monstrous, shrouded by time and secrecy.

When the war crumbled in 1945, Bayer did not recoil in shame. With the Third Reich's embers cooling, they crossed the Atlantic, their ambitions intact. In America, they unfurled a new banner: aspirin, a household name peddled as a shield against heart disease. But Bayer's gaze stretched beyond tablets. The same holding company, shadowed by whispers of eugenics a fixation not merely on Nazi ideology but on sculpting humanity to some twisted ideal began a quieter conquest: acquiring dairy farms across the United

States. Why dairy? The question gnaws like a splinter in the mind. By the mid20th century, Bayer's parent entities, linked to IG Farben (the conglomerate that fueled Hitler's war machine with Zyklon B), had dissolved their formal ties, but the ethos lingered. This was no random venture; it was a calculated expansion, a thread in a tapestry of control.

Bayer's agricultural arm, long intertwined with Monsanto a partnership formalized in their 2018 merger but rooted decades earlier moved in lockstep with its pharmaceutical sibling. Together, they lobbied the U.S. government with a fervor bordering on zealotry: "Make milk a cornerstone of every child's diet. Stockpile it transform it into cheese, powder, anything fortified with preservatives for longevity." The pitch was draped in patriotism: strong bones for a robust America. Campaigns like "Got Milk?" and the USDA's food pyramid, etched into schoolroom walls, sang dairy's praises. Milk, they insisted, was the elixir of health, a non- negotiable rite of childhood. Yet, as the decades rolled on, a grim harvest emerged. Children ballooned fat, lethargic, their bodies betraying them with chronic diseases: diabetes, asthma, allergies, conditions that didn't fade but clung like shadows. The dairy, laced with chemicals to sit on shelves for years, wasn't building strength; it was sowing sickness.

And who awaited with open arms? Bayer and its pharmaceutical kin, their labs humming with remedies not cures, but palliatives. Drugs flowed like rivers: treatments for inflammation, for insulin resistance, for the very ailments their dairy empire might have nurtured. The cycle was elegant in its brutality: feed the disease with one hand, medicate it with the other.

Profits swelled as the sick multiplied, tethered to prescriptions that dulled the pain but never severed its roots. Those Nazi experiments 300 women sacrificed cast a long shadow. What potions emerged from that carnage? Were they precursors to the biologics and stabilizers now ubiquitous, their origins scrubbed from public view? The files, if they survive, lie sealed, guarded by those who profit from silence.

This is no aberration; it's the pharmaceutical industry's grim refrain, a symphony of greed conducted across a century. Bayer's tale mirrors a broader legacy where profit eclipses life, and health is a distant echo. Take the Crohn's conspiracy, a microcosm of this ethos. Patients like Steve, ravaged by fistulas and inflammation, are handed biologics Remicade, Humira, Cimzia by Bayer and its ilk. These drugs, born of vast R&D budgets, douse the symptoms: the swelling, the pain, the endless fatigue. Yet, the root perhaps MAP bacteria, festering undetected remains untouched. Why? To cure is to lose a customer, to dry up the revenue stream. The inflammation, Steve argued, is the body's cry against infection, not a flaw to be silenced. But silence it they do, with immunosuppressants that list tuberculosis and cancer as side effects ironic, given Bayer's Naziera flirtation with such plagues. The patient lingers, a perpetual client, while the cause festers, profits assured.

History bears this out in blood and ledger ink. Merck's Vioxx, launched in 1999, masked arthritis pain but stopped hearts 50,000 dead by some estimates before its 2004 recall, all while raking in $2.5 billion annually. Pfizer's 1996 Trovan trials in Nigeria turned a meningitis outbreak into a laboratory, dosing children with an untested antibiotic; eleven died, dozens were maimed, and Pfizer settled for $75 million a pittance against their gains. Thalidomide, peddled by Chemie Grünenthal in the 1950s, promised serene sleep for pregnant women but birthed 10,000 deformed infants, its makers ignoring warnings for years to pad their coffers. Bayer's own Yaz contraceptives, aggressively marketed in the 2000s, triggered fatal blood clots in young women thousands suffered, yet sales hit $1.8 billion before scrutiny tightened. Each scandal reveals the calculus: treat the symptom, damn the source, and keep the cash flowing.

Bayer's journey from Nazi labs to America's dairy aisles to Crohn's wards embodies this creed. They bartered with genocide for science, flooded children with tainted milk, and now peddle palliatives to the chronically ill, all while the root causes rot in shadow. The industry thrives not on healing, but on sustaining sickness a machine oiled by human frailty, its gears grinding life into gold. From those 300 women to the millions tethered to pills today, the refrain endures: profit is king, and health, a disposable pawn.

Reflections

Medical Red Tape: The Clofazimine Crisis

Novartis was granted FDA approval of clofazimine in December 1986 as an orphan drug. The drug is currently no longer commercially available in the United States as Novartis has discontinued production of clofazimine for the US market and no generic or other brand names are marketed in the US although it retains FDA approval. Clofazimine, the generic name for the drug Lamprene, has not been available in US pharmacies since 2004.

This forced Steve to find alternative routes, ordering with a Canadian pharmacy that was importing the medication from India, where pharmacies sourced it from Abbott Labs in India.

Just as Steve began experiencing relief, a bureaucratic nightmare unfolded. The U.S. Food and Drug Administration (FDA) abruptly halted access to clofazimine worldwide, that I was getting from Abbott Labs in India. This happened during the questionable COVID19 pandemic.

Clofazimine, costing mere pennies per pill in India, had shown the potential to break down biofilms protective barriers that bacteria like MAP use to shield themselves from antibiotics. Removing access to this critical drug felt to Steve like more than a coincidence; it underscored what he saw as the "Crohn's conspiracy" a system unwilling or unable to pursue true cures due to regulatory hurdles, corporate interests, or a lack of financial incentive.

The Social Isolation of a Lifelong Battle

Throughout his thirties, Steve's relentless pursuit of answers came at a steep personal cost. His social world shrank as hospital visits, experimental treatments, and intense physical suffering consumed his daily life. Many of his peers couldn't comprehend the complexities of his illness or the sheer will it took to survive each day.

Yet, this isolation became a crucible for transformation. It was during these years of solitude and research that Steve's identity shifted from patient to advocate. He spoke at conferences, connected with scientists worldwide, and began educating others about the realities of living with Crohn's disease.

A Decade of Hard-Won Wisdom

By the end of his thirties, Steve's journey had reshaped not only his understanding of Crohn's disease but also his place in the world. He had exposed the cracks in a medical system ill equipped to handle chronic illnesses at their root and discovered alternative paths to relief when traditional medicine failed him.

His work became more than a personal quest it was a mission to challenge assumptions, demand better treatment options, and, above all, advocate for those too often ignored by the healthcare system. In this fight, Steve found not just survival but purpose.

Conclusion

Unbowed, Unbroken: The Fight Goes On

My journey with Crohn's disease has been a grueling marathon forty years of battling a relentless illness that claimed my mother's health, took my father at 26, and left me questioning whether I was fighting a genetic curse or a broken system. Through countless surgeries, shifting medications, and my own global research from the UK to India I've uncovered troubling patterns: a medical industry often more invested in managing symptoms than seeking cures, dismissive of dietary impacts I felt firsthand, and quick to push drugs that sometimes did more harm than good. This book, The Crohn's Conspiracy, isn't just my story it's a call to question, to dig deeper, and to reclaim control over our health.

I haven't found a cure. Complications from surgeries and the toll of past medications linger, and I still manage ongoing fistulas, with two or three flaring at any time. Yet, I've fought hard to avoid a colostomy bag and, in recent years, learned to handle my own care. In my thirties alone, I endured nearly a hundred trips to the operating room mostly for incision and drainage of fistulas leaving me so accustomed to sedation that no drug fully knocks me out anymore. Those years brought me to Dr. C, a rare surgeon who saw me as more than a case file. Patient and open, he taught me to maintain my fistulas without relying on biologic infusions, empowering me to take charge of my body before he retired. Without him, I might not be here, sharing this story.

Despite the scars, I've found ways to fight back closing a handful of fistulas over time, adapting my diet, and refusing to accept "incurable" as the final word. My hope is that this book lights a spark for you or a loved one, offering not just my truth but a path to question the system and explore what's possible; the fight continues. It will dive deeper into treatments, therapies, and emerging research like the role of Mycobacterium avium paratuberculosis (MAP) in Crohn's, colitis, IBD, and IBS. With new data and insights, my goal is to arm you with the knowledge to challenge the status quo and demand better. Here's to hope, resilience, and the truth.

X. Final Acknowledgements

Thank you to Dr. Maria for helping me get the triple antibiotic therapy and prescribed for the first time, Dr. Maria is a Brillant woman that made a treatment plan with Thomas Borody for me who helped me very much. Dr. Maria also helped me get Hyperbaric Oxygen Therapy which helped heal a lot of my infections at a time I was at my weakest.

Thank you to Dr. Saporta for always trying his best since a child to guide me in the correct direction. Dr. Saporta helped me when I needed prescriptions for the anti-map therapy when nobody else was willing

Thank you to Dr. Cohen Colorectal Surgeon for having patients with my fistulas and trying your very best at any technique or procedures we spoke about, thank you for all of the relief and sorry for all of the visits to the operating room. Glad you retired you deserve it! Thank you to Dr. Zanneti Hyperbaric Oxygen Therapy for believing in me and my research.

Thank you to Jason Page for taking the time and patience to talk to me and listen to my horrible story! Thank you, Jason, for all of your hard work, without you I would never have a book! You have always been a good friend and help, **Thank you**.

www.ingramcontent.com/pod-product-compliance
Lightning Source LLC
Chambersburg PA
CBHW062054270326
41931CB00013B/3070